It's Just Cancer

Making a Great Day, One Round of
Chemo at a Time
By: Brad Lubken

Published by Brad Lubken
Tacoma, Washington

This book is dedicated to my
family and friends who were
there for me in my greatest time
of need, and in honor of
Survivors everywhere.

Table of Contents

Preface

What This Book Is and Isn't

Before you read anything, make sure you know what you are about to get yourself into. I wrote this book for those who either have cancer, have a friend or family member with cancer, or in one way or another have been affected by cancer. I tell my story and what I experienced. Since each person's battle is unique, this book is not meant to be a guide to what will happen and how you should approach it. And, by no means is this book meant to be some sort of medical reference guide. Please, do not rely on my word alone. Your doctors are your biggest champions and best resources for questions.

I was diagnosed with cancer when I was twenty years old. Of course, I was scared to death, but I was also incredibly lonely because I didn't know anybody else my age who faced (or was facing) the same challenges I was. The isolation was unbearable. It is important to me that other young people have a resource to go to when they feel the need to relate. With that audience in mind, you will notice that as I tell my story I do so very candidly. At times I use somewhat vulgar language, am inappropriately honest, and make light of a very serious subject. Don't let that scare you away. My story is important to hear, and you will be a better person for reading it.

Last, this book is certainly not a literary masterpiece. Sure, I took the time to ensure I don't sound like a third grade dropout, but no professional editor was solicited to prepare this for publishing. I know there are plenty of areas which can be improved. But, since I want to get this book out to the masses and am doing so without the help of a publisher, you get to deal with that.

With that said, I hope you enjoy my book. It has been a labor of love which, from start to finish, has spanned eight years. Whether you are a survivor, currently in the process of surviving, or a supporter of a survivor, I thank you for purchasing this book and I wish you the best in all your life's battles. Make a great day!

Intro

Congratulations. Consider yourself lucky to be in the situation in which you have found yourself. I am assuming that you chose to read this book because you either have cancer, know somebody who has or has had cancer, or have been personally affected by cancer in one way or another. I say "congratulations" because I know through my experience with testicular cancer that cancer can actually be a blessing in disguise; if you choose for it to be so. Such a statement may sound radical now, but by the end of this book, I hope that you will agree with me. Buying into my story and learning from what I have learned will open doors you never imagined and make life a much more enjoyable adventure.

Cancer. Granted it's not the most fun thing to go through, but let me begin by saying there are plenty worse things one can experience. I say this because having gone through such an ordeal I know that honest reassurance is necessary to be able to confront the challenges that lie ahead. I decided to write this book because I felt that I had a story that needed to be shared so others can learn from my experience. I hope my story can both educate and comfort others who are forced to deal with the trials of cancer.

Part 1

1. *Before Cancer - Diagnosis*

Before It All Began

I made a hard turn to starboard (the right) and WHAM! The downrigger tripped and I had a 20lb king salmon on the other end of my line. "Holy shit!" I screamed. I didn't think of what I would do if I actually got a fish hooked. "How the hell am I going to reel in this fish?"

One month earlier I had ligament reconstruction surgery on my right wrist to repair two ligaments that had torn two years earlier during my senior year of high school. Somehow I still managed to work at a local pizza restaurant/brewery as a prep cook with one hand. Somehow I managed to drive my stick shift Mazda Miata around with one hand. Somehow I had managed to prep the boat and set all of the equipment to go fishing with one hand. But, how in the world was I going to bring in this fish?

Slowly (very slowly) I began to reel with the handle of the reel placed gently in-between my casted thumb and forefinger. My plan was to not fight the fish at all but to let it tire itself out and reel in the excess line hopefully without letting the hook slip out of its mouth. After several minutes of gaining ground on the salmon (all the while running back and forth to the steering console to turn the boat so the fish wouldn't tangle the line in the propeller) I finally saw the fish surface approximately twenty yards off the stern.

I turned to grab the net only to find I had left it in the boat locker. "Son-of-a-bitch!" I groaned. "I managed to reel in this beautiful salmon and I won't be able to bring it in the boat!" Realizing I had to get creative, I brought the fish up next to the boat, held the rod between my legs, knelt down, and reached my left hand fingers into the gills lifting the salmon into the boat. VICTORY!

I tell you this story because I realize it is an example of the fact that I am not the type of person to accept limitations. If I am told I cannot do something I am only driven further to triumph above that supposed constraint. Call it determination, fortitude, stubbornness, whatever. I have always known I have this trait about me but it wasn't until I faced cancer that I came to realize that my determination is exceptional; it is more the exception than the rule. My doctor told me that under no circumstances was I to be lifting anything with my right hand or to stress it in any way. But it was my day off of work and I wanted to go fishing. Sure, I wasn't supposed to do anything that could stress my wrist, but I wanted to go fishing; so I did. You think a little medical issue will get me down? Think again!

Allow Me To Introduce Myself

Hello, my name is Brad Lubken. Prior to July 30th, 2004 I was your typical college aged guy, facing typical issues faced by young adults, and anticipated leading a life one might consider more or less, well, typical. However, the journey I was about to take involved the most unexpected series of events that would forever change my life and consequently change myself and my life to be anything but typical.

Instead of jumping straight into my story of being faced with cancer, I'd like to begin by giving you a brief background of who I am. They say "you can't know where you are going unless you know where you've been". I want to introduce myself so you can learn how I became the person I was prior to cancer, and my intent is to share my story to explain who I have become having since survived cancer.

I was born on September 19th, 1983 in Tacoma, Washington to my parents Bill and Jean Lubken. I am the youngest of three children, with two older sisters. Our family of five lived in a suburb of Tacoma, known as University Place, until the three of us kids grew up and began lives and careers of our own.

My father was and continues to be a prominent periodontist (a gum disease dentist… or as I like to say, "the guy you really don't want to have to see, but you are happy he's around if you need him") with his office in Gig Harbor, Washington. He went to college for a total of nine years, as well as served in the United States Air National Guard for twenty years, retiring at the rank of Lieutenant Colonel. Throughout his career he has taught at local colleges, been elected President of the Pierce County, Washington State Dental Society, and has proved to be one hell of a dad.

My mother was and continues to be very active in the Washington State educational system. Throughout the years she has been a teacher, counselor, principal, and vice-principal across all grade levels. At the time of this writing she is working on earning her national board credentials; an accreditation which acknowledges teachers as the best of the best in education. Like my dad, she has also proven to be one hell of a mom.

My parents instilled the values of endless education, hard work, and perseverance in all three of their children. While being raised, we were always given quite a long leash where we were free to make our own choices all the while still being under their parental supervision. This allowed us to learn how to appropriately manage independence while forcing us to take responsibility for our actions. It is in large part to their approach to parenting that I grew to be the responsible "pre-cancer" me. However, it is also because of them that I was able to make what could have been seen as a tragic diagnosis into a life altering, wonderful learning experience. More on this later in the book.

Early in my adolescence I was very shy, reserved, and grew to develop seemingly low self-esteem. I remember times in middle school (fifth grade or so) when I would listen to music alone during recess, rather than play with the other kids, because I was afraid of fitting in with everybody else. God knows where this came from. Anybody who has ever met my mom knows it couldn't have been from her. I don't think she has any concept of timidity or self-doubt. My father has always been a bit reserved, but always made a point to be well educated so doubt would not interfere with your life. I chalk my self-doubt up to simply growing up and dealing with the societal issues we all deal with at that age. I only now realize that everybody else was probably feeling the same thing, only dealing with it in their own way.

While in junior high school I began to free myself from my self-imposed restraints and found myself growing more outgoing and therefore displaying much more confidence. I took part in student government and in high school I was constantly on stage performing be it acting, singing, or playing trombone in band. Get this. Four of my eight classes in my Senior year were performing arts classes: Symphonic Band, A'Cappella Choir, Swing Choir, and Advanced Drama. Oh yeah, I was also a starting lineman on the Varsity Football team. Every spring semester my favorite extracurricular activity was participating in the annual musical theater production. Can you tell I grew to not let societal norms restrict me? I suppose you could argue I even strove to break stereotypes.

I chose to attend my sister Andrea's Alma Matter for college; Pacific Lutheran University in Parkland, Washington. My main reason for attending PLU was to play football there and learn from a legend in his own right; coach Frosty Westering (I will talk about Frosty later). However, after finding two torn ligaments in my right wrist, and the two surgeries that followed, my collegiate football career ended before it began. In place of playing football, I auditioned for and received a vocal music scholarship singing bass and joined the choral program of the PLU music department. This turned out to be one of the best things that happened to me because of the people I met and the experiences I encountered.

Well, this brings me to the beginning of my story. When you flip the page the time will be late July of 2004. I will soon be entering my Junior year of college, my third year in the choral program at PLU, and my second year in the widely acclaimed Choir of the West. I will also be in the midst of my third year of coaching high school football (my second year coaching at the high school I attended, George R. Curtis Senior High School). I hope you enjoy reading what I experienced and learning why I say that cancer is the best thing to have ever happened to me.

● ● ●

Symptoms

I've always been a relatively tough guy. Being so tall (6'5") I often felt like being strong was expected of me. So when I first felt the throbbing ache in my right testicle, I blew it off as something that was no big deal. The pain was something best appreciated only by a member of the male gender. Ladies, use your imagination when reading the following. The pain felt as if somebody mildly flicked my right testicle. There was a combination of a continuous throb in my right testicle and an unsettledness in my stomach. "What the hell is this?" I asked as I adjusted myself assuming I was just sitting in such a position that was causing the uncomfortable tenderness. Realize that this pain wasn't excruciating or incapacitating in any way; it was simply a sore throbbing that caught my attention from time to time.

In addition to the pain, there was physical evidence that something may have been wrong; this too I chose to dismiss as something natural. When I looked in the mirror, I noticed my right testicle had grown noticeably larger than my left. This didn't concern me at all because a size difference had been the case all my life. I just thought to myself, "Huh! My right nut is a champ! Look how big it is." When I examined myself, I noticed that as my left testicle was smooth and soft whereas my right testicle had three distinct bumps and was comparatively harder than the left. For anybody else this should have been an immediate red flag and cause for concern; but, I had reason to dismiss this as well. Two years prior to this (the summer I graduated high school) I had a physical exam because I was training to play football at Pacific Lutheran University. While at that physical, I asked my doctor to check my right testicle because I felt what I thought was a bump. After examining me, he told me the bump I felt was actually my Epididymis (a hose like tubing in the scrotum that caries the sperm to the penis). It was simply a coincidence that I felt this "bump" on the same testicle two years prior to the concerns I am now describing. So, with the assurance that the "bump" I felt was normal, I dismissed these three bumps I most recently discovered.

Before Cancer - Diagnosis

Despite all the signs, I was now set on a course to completely overlook the possibility of having testicular cancer.

In addition to my enlarged and lumpy testicle, I had yet another (although less obvious) sign of some distress my body was experiencing. My family and I were driving from Tacoma, Washington to Clarkston, Washington (about a 6 hour drive) for a small family reunion. While on the drive, my right lower back began to ache. The aches were of little concern since such aches are common when crammed into a car with four other people. We stayed in a hotel for two nights before returning home. The pain continually increased as the weekend progressed and became unbearable on our way back home. I thought I must have aggravated my back on the uncomfortable pull-out bed I slept on in the hotel; so, once again I had reason not to be concerned of the pains I was feeling. As we continued home I was literally in tears due to the pain in my back.

Since I had it set in my mind that I somehow tweaked a muscle in my back, I arranged to have a massage to work out the knot and finally alleviate my horrendous pain. As I stepped into the building for my massage, I grew nervous because I never had a massage before. I didn't know what I was supposed to do. Was I wearing the right clothes? Was I supposed to bring anything with me? Do I wear clothes when I'm on the table? I didn't want to be laying naked on the table and have that be the wrong thing to do. I can just imagine myself being arrested for indecent exposure when all I want to do is to get rid of my back pain! Thankfully, I wasn't arrested, but when my massage was over, my back actually felt worse than when I went in.

Approximately one week later, my good friend Marisa and I went out to dinner at one of our favorite restaurants, The Olive Garden. I ordered the Tour of Italy which includes a lightly breaded piece of parmesan chicken. After a nice dinner we said goodnight and went to our respective homes. The next morning I headed off to The Rock, a local pizza place/bar, where I was a cook. I was cutting up vegetables preparing for the day's business when I suddenly began to feel nauseous and I sprinted into the bathroom where my suspicions of being sick were met with a lovely mixture of colors and consistencies of throw-up. My boss sent me home where I made an appointment with my family doctor later that day.

"I think I have food poisoning." I said. Ever since I was hired as a cook, I developed a paranoia concerning food safety. I told my doctor about the dinner I had the night before and stated that I believe the chicken was to blame for the sudden sickness I developed early that morning. He was about to leave the room to get his prescription pad to write me a prescription for some anti-nausea medicine when I quickly yelled, "Wait!" As the doctor returned I continued, "I've been having some pain... well... in my groin. Do you mind taking a look?" I never planned on asking him about the pain. The pain was so minute and inconsistent that I wasn't really concerned. But, since I was there, I figured I might as well get it checked out. After a few feels here and pokes there, my doctor declared, "You know this is probably nothing to worry about. There are some very evident lumps, but it very well may just be a cist, something very normal. These are common for guys your age. Let's order an ultrasound just to be sure it's nothing more than that." So there I sat. I just wanted to confirm the pain was nothing to worry about and instead, I headed out to schedule an ultrasound for a few days later.

I hid that my doctor wanted an ultrasound from my parents because I didn't want them to worry. I honestly wasn't that concerned because in my mind I accepted that the ultrasound was simply a precaution and therefore nothing to worry about. "Why worry them before we know if there's something wrong?" I justified. However, my parents did find out about my appointment preemptively because the reminder phone call came in when I was standing next to my dad in our kitchen. I tried to choose my words carefully so he wouldn't wonder who I was talking to, but I wasn't quite sly enough. "Who was that?" he asked. I paused for a quick moment interjecting a few uh's and um's, but I couldn't lie quick enough. I then began to tell my dad the whole story and from that point on the cat was out of the bag. All I could think was, "Let the worrying begin."

Diagnosis

An ultrasound of the testicles is the exact same as what pregnant women get to see their child in the womb. A gel is applied to the scanning area and when scanned, a real time image is seen on a monitor. You can think of the image like an x-ray in the sense that the image measures density. The harder the tissue the whiter it appears. Likewise, the softer the tissue, the more gray it appears. If any cancer is prevalent it would show as a white mass.

So I walked into the office for my ultrasound having no idea what to expect. My first feeling was embarrassment because although the people around me had no way of knowing why I was there, or what procedure I was having, I couldn't help but think everybody knew I was there for an ultrasound on my testes. In my head I could hear them laughing at the fact that something might be wrong with my junk. Every minute that passed was excruciatingly uncomfortable although I knew there was nothing to be embarrassed about. They didn't know why I was there, and even if they did, there is nothing shameful about taking care of yourself.

My name was finally called and I walked with a lady back to a room where I waited for the radiologist who was going to perform my ultrasound. Only a minute or two passed before an incredibly beautiful woman in her late twenties or early thirties walked in with two hand towels. She rolled one towel like a tube and kept the other towel unfolded. "Go ahead and take off your pants. Lie on the table and put the rolled towel under your scrotum and the open towel over your penis. I'll be back in a few minutes when you are ready." If the experience wasn't embarrassing enough, I now feel like a freaking science project! And, on top of that, it didn't help things that the radiologist was an attractive woman (for certain obvious reasons)... baseball, baseball, baseball.

Before Cancer - Diagnosis

I prepped myself and was left lying on the table until she came back into the room. She then applied a very thick layer of goo to both my scrotum and the sensor that performs the ultrasound. She moved the sensor around for what seemed to be forever but must have been only a few minutes. I could see the image on the screen out of the corner of my eye and I strained to try and make sense of what I saw, but my efforts proved worthless.

I had no idea what I was looking at. The image began as a grey scale picture which was what I expected. However, as time passed, the lady performing the ultrasound pushed a button and everything on the screen turned a different color. I can only assume it depicted varying temperatures because the colors reminded me of the weather section of a newspaper; blue for cold and red for hot. I couldn't reason how I could have such varying temperatures in such a limited area, and to this day I still don't know what all those colors were. As I continued to question what it was I was looking at, I was startled by an awkward loud grumbling noise coming from the machine. "What's that?" I asked. Evidently, it was yet another part of the scan I wasn't expecting

Once the sounds were turned off, she said the scan was over but she wanted another technician to take some pictures to be as thorough as possible. At that moment, my heart sunk and every conceivable thought flew through my brain. "I must have cancer if she wants a second opinion. But, maybe she's just being sure and doesn't see anything. But she's a qualified technician! The only reason she would have another person look would be if she was concerned about something! This can't be good." Although my thoughts were going into hysterics, I finally decided not to worry about anything because there was nothing yet to worry about. After the second person checked the images I wiped off the goo and drove home.

Only two days after my ultrasound I had an appointment with a Urologist to have the ultrasound read. It was Friday, July 30th. Before I continue, let me remind you that this doctor was a Urologist. Maybe it's just me, but I thought it was hilarious that his name was Dr. Wang (not pronounced "wong"). Honestly, if you want to become a doctor, that's great; but, if your last name was Wang don't you think you'd become anything besides a Urologist? But I digress. Dr. Wang entered the room with the ultrasound films in hand. I shook his hand and we both sat down.

I immediately grew uncomfortable because he presented himself with a very nervous demeanor. I figure he was a fairly new doctor and didn't know exactly how to deliver bad news. He rolled his chair uncomfortably close to me as an eerie silence filled the room. I felt like his nose was going to touch mine, he was so close. Nothing could have prepared me for what he was about to ask me. "So, uh, Brad. Do you ever want to have children?" was the first words out of his mouth. Caught off guard by the question I laughed and asked, "So, it's not good news, huh?"

His nervousness continued to show as he said, "I'm sorry, but I like to tell it how it is. I don't beat around the bush. You know? I'm a straight shooter and don't like to beat around the bush. I just like to tell how it is. I find that if you draw things out, people get more nervous. So, I just get things out in the open and tell it how it is. I just don't think it's a good idea to beat around the bush." Trying not to laugh as I listened to him try "not to beat around the bush," I assured him that it was okay and that his assertiveness didn't offend me.

He then showed me the films and to my amazement each picture of my right testicle was practically all white. You would have thought you were looking at a picture of a snowball. After explaining the films to me he finally said that yes I indeed did have cancer. Most people would think that hearing I had cancer would be pretty devastating news. But, for some reason unbeknownst to me, I took the news pretty much with a grain of salt. I wasn't really fazed at all by the news. As a matter of fact, I said, "Okay, so the first step would be to deposit sperm, right?" I think I surprised Dr. Wang not only because I knew I'd have to go to the sperm bank, but also by not sounding concerned. He must have thought I was taking it worse than I truly was because when he left the room to schedule an immediate appointment at a local sperm bank, a nurse came in, obviously for the purpose of consoling me, and making sure I was handling the news okay. She talked in a very soothing voice and made certain to never lose eye contact. The entire situation was extremely uncomfortable because it was like they were trying to make me feel bad about having cancer but I wasn't sad at all; granted I was probably in shock.

Dr. Wang entered the room once again and began to explain that it is vital to remove the testicle. I wasn't quite sure why it was such an urgent matter. All I knew was that it was cancer and that I didn't want cancer in my body. He didn't tell me why it was vital. Was it because the cancer could spread? Might the cancer make me sterile? I didn't know why it was so important to remove the testicle, but I remembered seeing a Tom Green Special on MTV about when he had cancer and his testicle was removed so I just figured that was common procedure.

Dr. Wang gave me two options, "We can take a biopsy of the testicle and see if it is malignant, but since most of the testicle is engulfed with cancer only a very little bit of testicle will remain and after losing so much of it, the remaining bit will most likely not function. If the cancer does turn out to be malignant, you will have to undergo another surgery to remove the rest of the remaining testicle. Or, we can go in and take out the entire testicle just to be sure we get it all. I would strongly suggest taking it all out, though." I said, "Take the whole thing. I don't want to risk it." He agreed that was the best decision and we scheduled surgery for his next available time, seven days later on Friday, August the 6th. I then left his office and drove myself to the sperm bank.

2.   *Sperm Bank - Orchiectomy*

So, This Is What A Sperm Bank Looks Like

Let me begin by saying if you have testicular cancer (or any kind of illness that may jeopardize your fertility for that matter), and you think you might want kids later on in life, don't allow anything to get in the way of depositing sperm. Whether it be a matter of pride, embarrassment, money, etc., you need to rise above any reasons against freezing your sperm and do it. Before you are cured of your cancer there will almost certainly be several instances when your fertility may seriously be put in jeopardy. You owe it to yourself, your partner, and your future children to be proactive and deposit. Even if you don't think you'll want children, you may decide later on that you do want kids and if you are not proactive about it immediately, it may very well be too late to potentially have children. Think of it like car or health insurance. You may not ever need to rely on it, but if you do need it, it is there for you.

I found my way to the sperm bank and was very apprehensive about going in. When I was in the parking lot, I didn't get out of the car immediately; rather, I sat there and took a few deep breaths before going in. For anybody, especially a first timer, a sperm bank can understandably be a very intimidating place. Honestly, where else do you walk in and you can't help but think the unsaid greeting to always be, "Hello. I'm here to masturbate into a cup. How are you today?" So I bit the bullet and went in. I was delightfully surprised to find a very welcoming/comfortable environment around me. Allow me to describe what the sperm bank experience was like.

After I took the elevator to the 3rd floor of the building (called the GYFT Clinic), I entered the reception area where there was a welcoming desk to check in at every visit. Here I simply notified the staff that I was there and made my way up to the 4th floor where the actual deposit site (sperm bank) is. The third floor is for Gynecology. Once on the 4th floor, I was handed a brown

● ● ●
13

paper bag which contained a sealed plastic cup in which I was to deposit my sperm. I was then assigned a room for privacy. In the rooms I found there were no videos to watch but there were adult magazines to look at. Unlike one of my favorite comedians Jeff Foxworthy, I didn't have to "use my imagination." There was also a very comfortable leather chair to sit in; but don't worry, each room is thoroughly cleaned after each person uses it. After ejaculating into the cup, the cup was sealed and placed back in the brown paper bag. Again, like Foxworthy says, "I like to wait a few minutes before I go out so I don't look like some kind of circus freak!" Lastly, I returned to the counter where I received the bag and handed my bag to the technician after filling out a survey which assists in analyzing the specimen. Once the process was over, I simply went on with the rest of my day.

After making my first visit to the sperm bank, I went to my dad's dental office to tell him the unfortunate news I received earlier that day. I asked his receptionist if I could talk to him and we went into his office where I told him my "adventures" I had that day. My dad, being in the medical field himself, was fairly calm and dealt rationally with the news. He began finding connections between the pains in my back and my diagnosis. Each detail I gave was met with a calm reaction which reflected both understanding and care. On the other hand, when I left the office and went home to tell my mother the news, she refused to accept that her only son and youngest of three children could have a life threatening disease. She turned frantic and immediately called some of her closest friends asking if they knew any good Urologists in the area; desperate for a second opinion. She also called who used to be my pediatrician, Dr. Ron Galucci. All of her sources referred her to one name; Dr. John Vaccaro. To try and calm and appease my mom, I agreed to be seen by him.

The Second Opinion

When she called Dr. Vaccaro's office, the receptionist informed us that there were no times available to be seen and that it was office policy to not offer second opinions. I can't figure out for the life of me why an office would not offer second opinions. As the receptionist listened to the panic in my mother's voice she calmly replied, "Listen, I'm a mother as well and I can only imagine what you must be feeling. How about this. Come in right now and I'll find a way to fit you in." So both of my parents and I headed off to Allenmore Hospital in Tacoma, WA where Dr. Vaccaro's office is located and we waited for him to be available.

After a very short wait I met with the doctor. Once again I was asked to take off my pants as he began to examine my testicle in question. Once he was finished examining me, he asked me to turnaround and put my elbows on the table. "Oh crap! I know where this is leading" I thought to myself. And sure enough, there went his fingers up my butt. And not only that; but he did it so hard that it hurt and it felt like he was trying to tickle my throat via rectum!

Dr. Vaccaro then allowed me to clean the lubricant off of me and get dressed as he said, "Yep! There is no doubt that this is cancer. There are three very noticeable bumps on your right testicle and it is also very large in comparison with the left." My right testicle was about twice the size of my left. He then invited my parents and me into his office where he explained the options from which I had to choose.

He first said it is important to have the infected testicle removed as soon as possible. When I told him I had an appointment with Dr. Wang one week later, Dr. Vaccaro became concerned. "I don't know of Dr. Wang and I wouldn't want to take a patient away from him, so the decision is ultimately yours; but I wouldn't like to see this postponed until next Friday because this is a very fast growing cancer. Testicular cancer can actually double in size in a matter of days. I would prefer to get you into surgery right now." I was shocked to hear how fast it could grow and that he wanted me in surgery so immediately. "Have you had anything to eat or drink in the last six hours?" he asked. "Look at me. I'm huge!" I said jokingly, "Of course I have." He said he could schedule me for surgery first thing Monday morning, but if I wished to keep the appointment with Dr. Wang, that was perfectly

● ● ●

15

fine. My parents and I discussed the options and we all agreed: since Dr. Vaccaro came so highly recommended and he can perform the surgery much sooner than Dr. Wang, we opted to have Dr. Vaccaro perform the surgery. No offense to Dr. Wang, but I also felt more comfortable with Dr. Vaccaro because he had considerably more experience.

As you can tell, I was faced with a difficult decision. How can I switch from Dr. Wang to Dr. Vaccaro? Politically this could very well cause friction between the two doctors. But what I realized is what I wish to pass on to you the reader. If you are faced with a life threatening disease such as this, you need not worry about more trivial issues such as what I dealt with. Think of it this way: it is your life that is threatened, you have the right to be selfish, and the most important aspect of treatment is feeling comfortable with that treatment. Never feel like you are stuck. If at any time you feel uncomfortable with your medical team, you have the right (duty in my opinion) to either discuss your troubles with your doctor(s) and/or find another doctor.

Surgery Number One: Orchiectomy

I waited for the weekend to pass and finally Monday came for me to go in to surgery. Sunday was very uncomfortable since you are not allowed to eat or drink anything 24 hours before your surgery, and my surgery was scheduled early in the morning. Most guys would think losing a testicle would be a painful experience. But the truth is that both the surgery and the recovery are relatively painless. The procedure is simple. An incision is made just below the waist on the side of the cancerous testicle. The surgeon then finds the Spermatic Cord that is connected to the testicle. Most people believe the testicles are freefalling, but there is a cord connected to each testicle which reaches up into your lower abdomen. The cord is then cut and the testicle is simply lifted out. The incision is then closed with a few staples (which are completely painless as well) and the heeling takes roughly one week. Even getting the staples removed after one week is painless. The only discomfort I felt was a tiny tug and maybe the slightest pinch when the staples were pulled out.

I woke up early on the morning of Monday, August, 2nd, 2004 when my mother drove me to Allenmore Hospital where my surgery took place. We entered the hospital and sat in the check-in waiting room; here you wait to give your insurance information, sign some release forms, etc. I noticed a woman in the room who smiled at my mom and me when we walked in and she began to walk towards us. I had no idea who she was and she was wearing some pretty odd looking clothes for being out in public. She was decked out in what looked to be a robe accessorized with a giant purple bow on the collar. It wasn't until she introduced herself, and I saw the crucifix necklace draped around her neck, that I realized she was the deacon from my church, St. Andrew's Episcopal.

After all my papers were signed the three of us sat down and talked as I waited to be taken to be prepped for surgery. We talked about my very fortunate diagnosis, any concerns I had (which were nil), and they both reassured me that everything would be fine. Again, I wasn't concerned at all about going into surgery, although I wasn't all that thrilled about losing one of my "boys". A nurse came into the lobby and called my name. It was time. The deacon said a quick prayer with my mom, dad, and me; then I left with the nurse to get ready for surgery.

Prior to surgery I was escorted to a changing room where I removed all my clothes, locked them in a locker, and put on one of those infamous surgical gowns that open in the back. (Get used to wearing these because you will be wearing them a lot for all of your surgeries and various medical scans.) I was also handed a pair of very ugly yet very comfortable ankle socks. Once dressed, I met with the anesthesiologist who inserted an IV into my right hand (get used to IV's as well) and explained what the drugs I would be given would do to me. Now that I was all prepped for surgery, I was escorted to the surgical room and placed on the surgical table. When the time came that the surgical team was ready, the anesthesiologist injected the drugs into the IV and asked me to count backwards from twenty. I began to count, "Twenty," I said confidently. "Nineteen," I said slurring. "Eigh…" and I was out. The instance right before unconsciousness sets in is the most euphoric feeling I've ever felt. My body turned numb and my mind clear. There was no fear about the coming incisions as all thinking seemed to seize.

The next thing I knew, I was unsuccessfully trying to open my eyes and make sense of what was going on around me. It's not the same activity as it was just a moment ago. As I tried and tried to open my eyes, I finally realized I was in the recovery room and the surgery was over. There was no perception of time as I swore that I was just about to begin surgery. A nurse approached me and asked how I felt. "I don't" I responded. I had yet to fully comprehend my surroundings as well as any sense of touch. She brought me juice and crackers until I had to ask her to stop.

I had a relentless call of nature and I needed to pee more than ever before. I asked the nurse where the bathroom was, expecting to go by myself. She called over a male nurse to help me to the bathroom because there was no way I was physically able to walk the few steps alone. He waited outside the door for me to finish and I knocked when I was ready for him to help me back to my bed. I was surprised that walking didn't hurt. I did have to walk hunched over slightly, but that was because the skin of my lower right abdomen was pulled tight by the staples. Be that as it may, I felt no pain whatsoever.

As far as the recovery is concerned, it was fairly painless. The worse part about it was the stretched area of stapled skin. Walking was not too bad of a challenge, I simply had to take small steps or else I would feel the staples pull. The only other challenge was keeping my dog off my lap because he loved to cuddle. As you can imagine, having him walk on my open incision wasn't the most comfortable feeling in the world. But, let me offer you some reassurance that this surgery is more of a minor inconvenience than anything else.

When we got the pathology report back (the post-surgical report that tells what the tumor cells consisted of), it was necessary

• • •

to find an Oncologist to administer the chemotherapy and/or radiation. The pathology report said that I have a type of testicular cancer that could only be treated with chemo; radiation therapy would not help. In fact, I was told that I just happen to be "lucky" enough to have the most aggressive type of testicular cancer there is. "That's a good thing?" I asked myself. There are evidently six types of testicular cancer, each having their own unique treatment. This most aggressive type of testicular cancer I had was the exact same type that almost killed the cancer advocate and world famous cyclist Lance Armstrong. We knew of an Oncologist who practiced in the Tacoma area and is always up to date on the latest cancer treatments. This doctor happened to be my fourth grade football team's team doctor. Dr. Vaccaro scheduled an appointment for me that Thursday with this doctor; Dr. Frank Senecal.

3.   *Beginning Chemo - Round 1*

Starting My Chemo Cocktail
Doctor's Notes

This is a 20 year old male patient who is a student at Pacific Lutheran University and presented his primary provider with complaints of stomach upset. He thought he maybe had food poisoning after eating at a local restaurant. He mentioned to his primary provider that he had been having some discomfort in his groin and wondered if he could examine the area. The area was examined and he was found to have a rock hard solid testicular mass on the right side. He was referred for ultrasound. The conclusion of the ultrasound revealed a well-circumcised mixed echogenic intratesticular mass measuring approximately 3.6, almost 4cm., in diameter. The differential diagnosis included non-aggressive germ cell tumor such as a dermoid. The possibility of a low grade malignant germ cell tumor cannot be excluded by this examination alone as well as neoplasm. He was then referred to Dr. John Vaccaro and the patient subsequently underwent a right testis and cord radical orchiectomy. The pathology reports revealed a mixed germ cell tumor with the following features: tumor included mature teratoma and embryonal carcinoma. Maximum tumor dimension was 4cm. Tumor was confined to the testes. No invasion of tunica albuginea identified. About the same time, the patient underwent a chest radiograph which was normal. He also had a CT of the pelvis and abdomen with the impression of a 5.4cm. retroperitoneal mass and a 6.1cm. right pelvic mass evident. The patient did have an alpha-fetoprotein drawn on 8/2/04 which was 2008.1. The patient is in today to meet with Dr. Senecal to review treatment options. The patient at this point is essentially asymptomatic except for some postoperative discomfort from his orchiectomy scar.

It was now the first Monday after my surgery, August 9th. I walked into the reception area of the office and I saw a group of people unlike any of group of people I had ever seen before. The majority of the people there were noticeably depressed, ill, and/or bald or thinning hair. I knew why these people looked the way they did, but it was a wake-up call to the fact that these people had cancer just like me; and the sight of them foreshadowed what I would look and feel like later on in my treatment.

My name was soon called and my mother and I were escorted to a private room where we waited to see Dr. Senecal. As time passed by while we continued to wait, our anxiety about what we were going to hear grew by the minute. The doctor was running behind at the time and we were waiting for about a half hour. Finally, Dr. Senecal walked through the door and almost immediately an unexpected calm doused our uncertainties. Dr. Senecal is a tall man with the most confident of swaggers. His love for his patients beams through his gentle eyes, his ever welcoming smile, and his oh so soft and caring voice. In addition, he keeps a cleanly shaven head in support of those he loves; his patients. It would be near impossible not to feel comfortable in his presence.

He sat us down and began to explain what steps should be taken in order to most successfully fight the cancer. He mentioned that my pre-surgical AFP, measured from blood I had drawn just before my orchiectomy, was at 2,008.1; drastically above a normal level of 6. My post-surgical AFP was measured at 802. During our conversation, he included that with this type of cancer, at my age, and in my health that I had a 99% chance of cure. I felt an incredible sense of relief the moment I heard this fact. He advised that starting the next week, I check into St. Joe's Hospital for five days and begin chemo where any adverse reactions could be monitored. I'm not sure if this is a normal thing to do when one begins a chemo regimen, but Dr. Senecal wanted to make sure all things went well with the drugs I was going to be given.

"What I need you to do is stop by the infusion room and show the nurses your chart" said Dr. Senecal. My mom and I went to the infusion room where we were told I was going to be given a dose of Bleomycin (Blee-o-mice-in). Bleomycin (known as Bleo) is a chemo therapy drug that I was given once a week throughout my treatment. We had no idea that I was going to begin my chemo therapy regimen that day, but I figured, "Why not start now? I'm

* * *

here. Let's do it." An IV was placed in a vein on top of my right hand and I only had to wait about twenty minutes for the Bleo to finish dripping into my blood stream. The nurse then removed the IV and I went merrily on my way. Believe it or not, from the first doctor's appointment I had due to food poisoning, to this my first "taste" of chemo, was only a period of seven days.

Doctor's Notes

Dr. Senecal met with the patient and his parents. He spent a good deal of time explaining the etiology of the disease and the treatment options available. Dr. Senecal feels that treatment should be started promptly and further evaluations should be done promptly. All the patient and family's questions were answered. Dr. Senecal discussed the pros and cons of chemotherapy. Also discussed the process of staging the disease and would like to make the following recommendations: 1) Repeat alpha-fetoprotein 2) also beat HCG, LDH, and chem-12, 3) PET scan to be done ASAP, 4) Send for pulmonary function test, 5) He will also be set up for a brain MRI at TRA which will be done this afternoon. Dr. Senecal also discussed initiating the first chemotherapy in the hospital and this will probably take place this coming Wednesday when he will have a PET scan done. The chemotherapy agents to be used will be Cisplatinum, Bleomycin, and VP-16.

Some people might think that once you begin chemo (injecting poisons) you would start to feel sick right away. The truth is that I felt just as good after I received the Bleo as I did before. There was no immediate affect from the chemo.

Per Dr. Senecal's orders, I had a Positron Emission Tomography (PET) scan conducted on my entire body to see if I had any cancer throughout the rest of my body. A PET scan is different from an MRI or a CT scan in that it is able to detect malignant or benign disease by injecting radioactive glucose into the bloodstream. If a tumor is active (cancerous) it absorbs the glucose. The PET machine (which looks almost exactly like a CT machine) has cameras which record the gamma rays emitted from the glucose and generate a corresponding medical image. Tumors are seen as areas of increased uptake because they absorb more of the glucose than the rest of your body.

Having a PET scan is a fairly easy process. I was given food options to eat the day before my scan. I was only allowed to eat low carbohydrate and/ high protein foods, so I decided to treat myself to a steak for dinner. However, I was not allowed to eat within six hours of the scan. My scan was scheduled for three o'clock the next day and since I accidently slept in that morning, I had nothing to eat all day. I was starving! When it was time for my scan there was an IV placed in my hand and the glucose was injected. One of the side effects of the solution was that it made me have to pee every ten minutes or so. They placed me in a dark room where I was told to rest for one hour so the glucose could spread throughout my body. Conveniently, I was sitting very close to the restroom. After the hour passed I was directed to the PET scanner which scanned my entire body in approximately forty-five minutes. Besides being hungry, the process was completely painless.

Dr. Senecal wanted me to get in to the hospital as soon as possible so I could begin my first of three planned rounds of chemo therapy. I was relaxing at home when I received a call from the hospital confirming that Dr. Senecal had requested a room for me, but they said they had no bed available for two days and they were trying to get a hold of my doctor to let him know as well. I didn't think much of it and figured it couldn't hurt to wait another two days. However, Dr. Senecal evidently thought otherwise.

Later that night I got another call from the hospital saying that they may have a bed open later that night in a different area of the hospital and they wanted to know how late they could call to ask me to come in. I let them know that I was willing to check in at any time, but I couldn't help but laugh at the fact as to how powerful Dr. Senecal's word was. Honestly! There was no bed open for at least two days, and once Dr. Senecal talked to the hospital they bent over backwards to get me in A.S.A.P. Be that as it may, the hospital was not able to get me in that night. Instead, they had me check in the very next morning at 8:00am.

After a restless night of sleep, I hopped in the car as my mother drove us to St. Joseph's Hospital in downtown Tacoma, Washington. Up until that moment I had yet to be concerned at all about what I was about to go through, and I continued to be very strong until the hospital was in sight and a certain song came on the radio station we were listening to. The song "You Raise Me Up" by Josh Grobin came on and my eyes gently began to fill with tears. I began to cry silently and I could not understand why I was doing so. It was the first time I became emotional over having cancer. Until then I was very positive and nonchalant. Little did I know that it was the first of several instances my emotions would get the better of me.

"Why am I crying?" I asked myself as I carefully wiped away my tears so my mom couldn't tell I was crying. Although I tried to justify my tears, I didn't understand why I was crying for quite some time. I now realize that seeing the hospital in the distance paired with the lyrics of the song that just came on the radio finally forced me acknowledge that my life was threatened and I actually had cancer. Read the lyrics of "You Raise Me Up;" it should help you appreciate the way I felt. It gave me hope as well; telling me I could beat this disease, building strength along the way. It was like a prayer from me to God, begging for His help as I began a journey I knew would change my life forever.

When I am down and, oh my soul, so weary;
When troubles come and my heart burdened be;
Then, I am still and wait here in the silence,
Until you come and sit awhile with me.

You raise me up, so I can stand on mountains;
You raise me up, to walk on stormy seas;
I am strong, when I am on your shoulders;
You raise me up... To more than I can be.

You raise me up, so I can stand on mountains;
You raise me up, to walk on stormy seas;
I am strong, when I am on your shoulders;
You raise me up... To more than I can be.

There is no life - no life without its hunger;
Each restless heart beats so imperfectly;
But when you come and I am filled with wonder,
Sometimes, I think I glimpse eternity.

You raise me up, so I can stand on mountains;
You raise me up, to walk on stormy seas;
I am strong, when I am on your shoulders;
You raise me up... To more than I can be.

You raise me up, so I can stand on mountains;
You raise me up, to walk on stormy seas;
I am strong, when I am on your shoulders;
You raise me up... To more than I can be.

You raise me up... To more than I can be.

Chemo Round Number 1

Now in the reception area of the hospital, I signed everything I needed to sign (insurance info, medical releases, etc.) and we were escorted to one of the top floors of the towering hospital. I was anxious to begin my chemo as soon as possible. "Let's get this party started," I thought to myself "the sooner we begin, the sooner I'll be cured." As I'm sure you can imagine, I was upset that all I did for the first two hours was sit and watch TV once I got settled in my room.

Finally, after two very long hours, a short man with a bushy graying beard approached me pulling a large computer on wheels behind him. I didn't know what the machine was for, but I soon discovered that this man was here to perform a spirometry test which measured how much air my lungs could inhale and exhale. "Take the biggest breath you can and blow as hard as possible into this tube. There is no backing on the tube, so it will feel as if you aren't blowing very hard, just do the best you can" said the doctor.

To give you a better idea of what the machine was like, imagine a pipe. This pipe is about five or so inches long and one inch in diameter. Both ends of the pipe are open and a hose is connected below the pipe through a third opening leading into the computer. At first glance this is a very odd looking, very complicated piece of machinery. This was an older machine so it was fairly large. More modern spirometers are small enough to fit in the palm of your hand.

I grabbed the tube, took a deep breath, and blew until the doctor said to stop. As I blew I watch the computer screen which displayed a graph of my blow in real time. There was a steep incline, a short plateau, and a sharp decline in the graph. "Ok, let's do it again, but his time really blow hard." I took a deep breath and blew until no air was left in my lungs to blow. The graph looked the same to me but the doctor said I did much better. "Alrighty, one more time as hard as you possibly can." For one last time I inhaled deeply and blew as hard as possible. This third and last blow was the best of the three. It was awkward to blow with a lot of strength because there was no resistance to blow against. You have to keep blowing even after you think your lungs are completely exhausted of any air. After each blow my head ached a little and I got slightly light headed, so don't worry if that happens to you as well; it's normal.

Once that test was over (all five minutes of it) I waited for about another hour for some ladies to come by to place something called a PICC-line (pronounced "pick-line") in my arm. I was told that having this "Peripherally Inserted Central Catheter" in my arm would make it so I wouldn't need to be poked with needles every time I get drugs. I thought this sounded like a great idea since I preferred not to get stuck with needles over and over and over again.

Two ladies, who looked to be in their mid-sixties, entered the room and told me that they were going to place an IV like tube in my right arm in the artery between my bicep and tricep. "Will

● ● ●

this hurt at all?" I asked. "Oh, no. We will numb your arm before we poke ya." she confided. The next thing I knew the entire room was flooded with blue tarp like towels. These blue "drop cloths" are all sterile and they are used because a sterile environment is necessary when putting in a PICC-line. Even the nurses were covered in blue.

The first step in the process of placing a PICC-line is finding the artery. To do this, the artery is found via ultrasound. Through the pictures, the nurses measure how deep the artery is in your arm, and in my case the artery was measured at 2cm deep. Next, the area is numbed as deep as the artery lies so the patient's pains are eased. This is a fairly painless part of the process. It's the equivalent of getting a flu shot. Lastly, the PICC-line is inserted by threading the line into the arm through the artery and is stopped once the end of the line lies up underneath your collar bone.

So, after they measured my artery at 2cm into my arm and numbed the area, they proceeded to insert the pick line. A moment went by and I thought nothing had happened yet. "Ok, we're almost to the artery" said one nurse. The next thing I knew I was gritting my teeth in pain as I could feel the line prodding at my artery wall, trying to break through. "Can you feel that?" questioned the nurse puzzlingly. I tell people it felt and heard like a screw drilling into concrete. She said I'd have to deal with the pain until they were done because it would hurt more to start over after injecting more anesthesia. Evidently, what happened was that they measured my artery at 2cm deep when it was actually 3cm deep. The pain was horrendous. In fact, I was so surprised by the immense pain that I began to feel a bit lightheaded. I got over the pain soon enough, but it was something I did not expect at all.

Now that the PICC-line was inserted, I had a tube dangling out of my right arm approximately two inches long along with two other tubes coming out of the main tube another six inches long. Once again, the purpose of this pick line is to administer the chemo drugs into my body without excess poking with needles. I knew the line was to make things easier for me, but then I was paranoid that I'd catch it on something, the line would pull out, and blood would fly around everywhere! Thank God that never happened, but it was just another concern to weigh on my mind which I certainly didn't need.

Doctor's Notes

An AP erect exam shows the tip of the PIC catheter is in the mid to distal SVC at the level of the right main stem bronchus. Cardiopulmonary appearance is normal.

"What do you do when you are in the hospital getting your chemo?" is a question I get quite a bit when I tell people I was in the hospital for five days. There really isn't much to do in the confines of a hospital bedroom. The first "exciting" thing I did while in the hospital was to pee in a measuring cup; trust me, it's just as glamorous and thrilling as it sounds. Every time nature called, I had to pee in to a large plastic measuring cup the resembled the container for a quart of milk. The nurses had me do this the entire time I was admitted to the hospital because they wanted to make sure that the amount of liquids exiting my body corresponded with the amount of liquids they put in my body.

Secondly, I was proactive to coming to the hospital by bringing an arsenal of DVD's with me to fill the void of boredom. Euro Trip, The Best of Will Ferrell and Adam Sandler from Saturday Night Live, Training Day, and plenty of other movies helped me pass the time in-between each urinary pit stop. Having a vast array of movies was great; however, the problem with movies is that once you watch a movie once, watching it again so soon almost became a chore rather than a fun way to pass the time.

In addition to movies, the TV in the room was a godsend. I am a TV junkie and love watching sitcoms, reality shows, and especially the news. (I know, I'm such a nerd!) Normally this would keep me occupied but I was just "lucky" enough to be in the hospital during the first week of August, 2004. That's right; this is right at the start of the Summer Olympics. Since the Olympics were in full swing, almost everything I got to watch mentioned them in one way or another. NBC was covering the games, so I couldn't watch any my favorite TV shows on that network; and every other channel had interviews with the athletes, news coverage of the games, or some other programming based around the Olympics which I was certain was scheduled for the sole purpose of pissing me off.

I also brought a copy (one of many I received since I was diagnosed) of Lance Armstrong's book It's Not About the Bike. I planned on reading bits of the book when all else failed to hold my interest. No offence to Lance or his book, but I'm just not the biggest fan of reading for fun. The first day I was in the hospital my mother couldn't put the book down and therefore I didn't have the opportunity to read any that first day. She loved the book so much that she managed to read the entire thing while we waited for everything to happen: the tests, my PICC-line, the chemo. Although I did have the book at my disposal, I did not read a single page during my stay at St. Joe's Hospital.

Most importantly I had friends and family constantly visiting me, wanting to keep my spirits up although I was very positive throughout the entire process. My parents visited me every day; usually together, sometimes separately, but nonetheless they were there every day. I believe it was the third night in the hospital when they arrived one night with a fresh–out-of-the-oven large pepperoni and sausage pizza from Round Table Pizza in hand. Once I saw my parents outside my door window with that pizza, all my bed fatigue disappeared instantly. It's funny how when you are placed in an unfamiliar/unforgiving space such as a stark white hospital room, something as familiar as your favorite pizza from your favorite pizza restaurant can let you feel like nothing is wrong and everything is as normal as it always is. You feel as if you are safe in the confines of your home simply eating dinner.

A visitor I had every day I was in the hospital was a friend from college; Helen. Helen is a girl I met through a mutual friend at Pacific Lutheran University (PLU). She was previously affected by cancer because her grandfather was diagnosed with cancer a few years before me. On her first visit, she brought me the LIVESTRONG bracelet (the well-known yellow fundraising bracelet of the Lance Armstrong Foundation) she wore when her grandfather had cancer that I still wear to the date of this writing. I also remember one visit when she brought me fresh picked blueberries from her grandmother's garden. "They're filled with antioxidants... my grandpa ate them all the time when going through his treatment" she said. I ate those berries as fast as I could, willing to try anything to help me beat my cancer. Helen would visit me alone, with her little sister, or with her mom so there was always something new to talk about. I can't thank Helen enough for being such a wonderful friend in my most needy of times.

I had a very unexpected visitor one day; my former priest Father West Davis. I was sleeping with the chemo drugs dripping into my arm when I barely cracked my eye open and noticed somebody sitting in the chair next to me. The sunlight glared my vision, but once I was able to focus my eyes I saw the face of my beloved retired priest whom I hadn't seen for years. We sat and talked about how I was diagnosed, my spirits, and life. Like everybody else, I reassured him that I was taking everything in stride and feeling just as positive as ever, if not more so. I talked to his daughter (my God Mother) Jeanine when she visited me at my parent's house after my orchiectomy and I assume it was through her that he found me at the hospital. Before he left, we both closed our eyes and bowed our heads as we held hands and he said a prayer for my well-being. As we prayed, he anointed my head with oil. "Amen" we said in unison. "You know... this is the same oil I used to baptize you when you were a baby." With a mutual sense of calmness, we said our goodbyes and once he left the room a single tear formed in my right eye and it fell down my check, landing on my arm.

Stephanie Johnson, another wonderful friend from PLU, visited me on her own one day. She knocked very softly on my room door and came in, peaking around the door not wanting to feel like an intruder. An uncontrollable smile came upon my face when her overwhelming personality filled the room. Steph is an amazingly talented singer/guitarist/entertainer with a sense of humor everybody can love. If you ask her for honesty, she'll give it to you straight. If she knows you need a pick-me-up, she's the first to give you the warmest, most sincere hug you can imagine.

As she came in the room I saw she had a bag full of things to keep me occupied while in the hospital. The bag included a bunch of magazines, an activity/puzzle book, and a CD of her music. Somehow she knew exactly what a guy in the hospital needed. She sat in a chair next to my bed and we talked for some time. Every so often I caught her eyeing the tubes from my body to the bags containing my chemo drugs. There was no need to say anything. I could understand her concern and questioning what I was going through. I just lay in bed and enjoyed every word we exchanged.

Another group of guests I received one day were my roommates from the prior year at college. Marisa, Brittnee, and Arynn came to visit me and it made me feel like we were all back in our town house just off campus again. Brittnee is the mother of the group. Her nurturing demeanor is undeniable and her maturity beyond her years is something I will always respect. Arynn is a firecracker of a blonde. She is outspoken, hilarious, and the girl that when she walks in to a bar all the guys' (and most the girls' for that matter) heads follow her in. I have already introduced you to Marisa, and you will get to know her a bit more throughout the book.

They sat in chairs around the bed and on the side of the bed itself as we talked about how I was feeling, what it's like to be in the hospital, and what I do to fill my time. The typical talking points as I came to know them. Britnee was a bit quieter than I knew her to be. In retrospect, it made sense being that she is the motherly type and was likely so taken aback by the sight that she was trying to find the right words to say; even though any words would have been the right words.

In typical Arynn fashion, Arynn said, "Ok, wait. So, they took one of your balls?"

"Yup" I replied. I would normally be taken aback by such a question, but not since it was coming from Arynn.

"Well, aren't you worried about what a girl might say or think when she is 'with' you?"

After laughing a bit as I could understand her question I said, "Well, if she doesn't like what she sees she can drive to Allenmore Hospital, find my removed nut, and suck it!" I absolutely understood Arynn's question, but when it comes down to it, if a girl has a problem with my post-cancer body that is her problem, not mine. I'd be better off without her.

I loved having my three girls come and visit me in the hospital. I'm pretty certain they still don't have any idea how much it meant for the three of them to be bedside and make me feel as if we were still in our house together; to make me feel like it was just like any other day.

Of course, the nursing staff was always by my side. When you are in the hospital, take advantage of the nursing staff there. The men and women there chose nursing as a career because they sincerely care and want to help people and comfort those in need; let them. There were times when a nurse came in to measure my urine, see if I was feeling nauseous, administer my chemo, and would just strike up a conversation because I was so bored of doing absolutely nothing. They truly did treat the patient rather than the disease, which is something I will always appreciate.

I'd talk to nurses at all times of the day: morning, afternoon, evening, night. But what I did find was that if I was awake during the graveyard shift (like 2:00am) those nurses loved to talk to you because nothing was going on in this area of the hospital at that time. I'm sure the Emergency Room was busy at that time of night, but where I was, the nursing staff had to sit in the dark and keep quiet for the sake of the sleeping patients.

I remember the day I was finally allowed to leave the hospital. My dad picked me up from the hospital and it felt absolutely amazing. Walking further than the distance from the bed to the bathroom, my legs could stretch. Breathing fresh air, I smelled scents other than stagnant stale hospital air. Eating at home, the food didn't taste like it was mass produced and simply warmed up for consumption. The friendliness of your own home, you don't feel like a patient any longer. It's like they say, "There's no place like home."

Doctor's Notes

The patient is a very pleasant gentleman, a 20-year-old that I saw the day before yesterday. Dr. Vaccaro was his Urologist. He was found to have a testicular mass on the right side, which was resected by a radical orchiectomy approach by Dr. Vaccaro. His CT scans demonstrated retroperitoneal adenopathy on the right side. Additionally, the patient had a cystic-like process in the right groin. Subsequent workup indicated an alpha-fetoprotein in the area of 10,000 with normal beta-hCG and an LDH that is pending at this point. We have placed him in an intermediate risk category. We plan on preceding with Cisplatinum, V-16, and Bleomycin chemotherapy tonight. His renal function is normal.

He was admitted to receive conventional therapy for this disease. He was treated with Cisplatinum 20/m sq. per day that is 47mg x 5 days, VP-16 at 100-mg/m sq. per day x 5 days, and Bleomycin as a single dose at 30 units. He tolerated this well. He did have some nausea and was given antiemetics including Amend x 3 days, Decadron, Ativan, and Kytril. He seems to be doing reasonably well.

4. *Surgery Number 2 - A Change of Plan*

Surgery Number 2: Port Placement

I was very lucky compared to many other chemo patients because I never got sick from my first cycle of chemo. I did feel the slightest bit nauseous from time to time, but that was the extent of it. Some people will have horrible reactions to their chemo drugs; nausea, vomiting, and sometimes (through extremely rare) even potentially fatal reactions to the chemo therapy. If such vicious reactions occur, they usually only happen on your initial cycle of chemo because your body does not appreciate having poison in it. Once the initial sickness is over, most patients' bodies adjust to the drugs and they tend to feel relatively okay (with the exception of the normal illness from prolonged exposure to chemo therapy; such as nausea, vomiting, etc.; which can be pretty horrible in their own right). If the adverse reactions continue, the doctor may opt to change the chemo regimen (or "cocktail" as chemo recipients tend to call it), switching the nauseating drug with another that may be gentler on the patient's body.

The next week I went to a checkup appointment at Dr. Senecal's office. I had to do a lab which reported my CBC and AFP (Complete Blood Count and Alpha-Fetoprotein). If you'll recall, my AFP previous to my first chemo cycle was 802; now, only after one week of chemo, my AFP count was at 84.9. Alpha-fetoprotein is something that everybody has in their body, but we should have a count of six or below. Anything above that is cause for concern. Pregnant women get a large increase of their AFP, but this is the only case (that I know of) when an increase of AFP is normal and healthy.

My family and I were very happy to hear that the chemo was doing its job, and so quickly too. However, there was still plenty of living cancer inside my body. Even though the chemo had begun killing the cancer, I was nowhere near finished or in the clear. Dr. Senecal checked my heart, lungs, and poked my abdomen as he had in my previous appointment. My check-up was

• • •

just about over when he said, "So we don't turn you into a human pincushion, we might want to consider having a port installed in your chest." He proceeded to describe what a port is and why I might want one. We then scheduled the surgery to install the port for the next Friday and left the office.

A port is a metal ring approximately an inch in diameter with a long catheter attached. The port was placed just below the collar bone on my right pectoral muscle and the catheter was threaded through my jugular artery until it reached my heart. This allowed the chemo to enter my body through the heart, which is very strong in comparison to the veins in my arms and hands. In addition to sparing yourself from countless needle-sticks, having a port eliminates the collapsing of veins which can happen when a vein is punctured too many times. The only evidence of anything foreign in your body is a circular lump under the skin where the metal ring is anchored.

It was Friday, August 27th and I was about to get my port installed. The surgery is typically only about a half hour to one hour long at the most. My mother drove me down to St. Joe's Hospital where I checked in and was whisked off to prep for my very simple surgery.

The process for prepping for surgery is roughly the same for each surgery. I was sat down in a room where there were other people preparing for surgery as well. I was asked to change into the ever so famous surgical robe that leaves your butt flying in the wind and I did so. Luckily, this surgery wasn't going to happen "downstairs", so I was allowed to keep my pants on. The nurse then took my vital signs (blood pressure, temperature, pulse, and respiratory rate) and said, "In just a few minutes the anesthesiologist will be in to talk to you" and I was left alone in my mildly uncomfortable chair.

In walked a tall man with several items securely wrapped to be sterile and he pulled over a rolling tray on which to place the items. He introduced himself and began to tell me what he was going to be doing to me. Because I have had surgeries prior to this, I already knew what to expect; but, for the sake of information

Surgery Number 2 - A Change of Plan

I will describe what the anesthesiology experience was like. The doctor placed an IV by inserting a needle into my right arm. Once the needle was in, what I would describe as a catheter (although I'm not sure if it is or not) also went into my arm and the needle was removed. Now, only the catheter is dangling out of your arm. The catheter was then connected to another tube which was connected to a bag of saline. Saline is basically salt water and is used for several purposes; in this case to dilute the drugs that were going to knock me out and to keep me hydrated.

The saline slowly dripped into my bloodstream until the surgical room and surgical staff was ready for me. A nurse then escorted me into the very intimidating surgical room. The grotesquely clean room had a table placed in the middle that looked like it is used to restrain mental patients. I laid on the hard, flat, metal table, which was covered in sheets, and warm sheets were placed on top of my shivering body. Finally, the moment of truth arrived and the anesthesiologist entered the room that saying he was going to put me under. As the anesthesia was injected into my IV, I asked, "Where are we going?" because I noticed the ceiling was moving and the table was rolling backwards. "We're about to begin surgery" explained a nurse. "Yeah I know" I said in a groggy voice, "but where are we moving to?" I knew the drugs were kicking in because the nurse replied, "Brad... you aren't moving."

"Now, begin counting backwards from twenty," ordered the anesthesiologist.

Whereas in my orchiectomy I managed to count half way through eighteen, I was determined to stay awake longer this time. I was making being put under a game. Hey, you've got to do something to make these painful experiences at least a little bit entertaining. I began, "Twenty, nineteen, eighteen, (I did it!) seve..." I was then in a deep, deep sleep.

One of the most surreal moments of the entire experience was waking up in the middle of the surgery and feeling the surgeon hitting my chest. I was lying on the table when my eyes opened and I could only see the familiar blue sterile sheets, but this time

* * *

they were over my head. I couldn't seem to move my body, but I could tell that I was in the middle of surgery. I felt a forceful rocking motion and realized the doctor was wailing on my chest where the port was to be installed. All I was capable of thinking was, "Why is he hitting me?!?!" And as soon as I woke up, I felt back asleep. I'm sure what I woke up to was not the surgeon hitting me, but simply doing what he needed to install the port. I'm certainly not trying to accuse my surgeon of assault.

"What is that sound? It doesn't sound like medical staff. Why can't I open my eyes? Oh, well, it doesn't matter. I feel incredible. What? Did somebody ask me something? It's my mom!"

I was in the recovery room and my mom was sitting in a chair next to my bed talking to me. I remember trying to respond, but whatever it was I said sounded like a Cro-Magnon grunt. I wasn't alert enough to actually talk yet. When I began to show signs of life, a recovery nurse (who happened to be a friend of my mom's) approached me and asked how I was feeling, if I felt nauseous, if I wanted anything. She left and returned with some juice and crackers that I had to down before I was allowed to go home. I have no idea why crackers and juice are always what is given to you after something medical; donating blood, donating plasma, coming out of this surgery, etc. If anybody knows why this is the case, I'd love to know. My theory is that it is some superstitious thing among nurses. Yep; that's the best I got.

Doctor's Notes

Fluoroscopic spot film demonstrates satisfactory position of right internal jugular chest port with catheter tip in superior vena cava at the cavoatrial junction. Catheter measures 20cm in length.

The Monday after I got out of the hospital from my first round of chemo, I went back to Dr. Senecal's office for my weekly dose of Bleo. Every Tuesday I was to show up to his office and get a small "baggie" of Bleo which, if you remember, took about twenty minutes to completely enter my body. This was my first opportunity to test out my recently installed port. I walked into the infusion room and grabbed a seat in one of the many large, very comfortable chairs. "Can you pull down the collar of your shirt so I can see the port, Brad?" asked the nurse. I exposed my new "jewelry" and she reached for a brown canister. "Brace yourself, okay? This won't hurt, but will be very cold on your skin." She sprayed what I learned was a lidocaine spray on the area of my port. It felt like ice. It was so cold that it almost felt like my skin would burn. To make sure the port would not back-up, saline was injected, leaving a salty/metallic taste in my mouth and an unpleasant smell in my nose. She then asked me to take a deep breath; and as I did, she pushed in an "L" shaped needle with an IV line connected at its end. The end of the IV line is then connected to the main IV and the drugs and saline drip slowly into your blood stream. Once all the Bleo was in, the nurse removed the needle from my port, covered the port with a Band-Aid, and I carried on with the rest of my day.

Doctor's Notes

The patient has started chemotherapy. He has received 1 cycle and will receive cycle 2 this week of platinum, Etoposide, and Bleomycin. Laboratory work is ordered. We will recheck alpha-fetoprotein. It will be our plan to repeat CT scan prior to cycle 3 of a planned 4 courses. Today, no neuropathy. Port was placed and has caused some discomfort, we will treat with Vicodin. I believe that some of this is due to a skin reaction he had due to the tape.

Chemo Round Number 2

The next Monday (August 30th) I went back to Dr. Senecal's office to begin yet another week of intensive chemo; my second round. On this the first of another five days of chemo, three vials of blood were drawn from my port and tested. They tested my CBC and AFP again and I found that my CBC showed 12 out of 31 criteria were abnormal and two others were close to being out of an acceptable range. It was my first wakeup call that the chemo was not only killing the cancer, but it was also killing me! I didn't receive the results of my AFP because it takes approximately two days to get those results back. Once the blood was drawn, I was ready to get my first of the three drugs I got that day (Bleo, Cisplatinum, and VP-16); but, as I would begin every day of chemo, I first had to receive a bag of saline for the purpose of staying hydrated. Once the saline was in, I got the other three drugs one at a time and finished with another bag of saline. The entire process took about five hours per day. But what does one do all that time? I won't glorify anything. It was very boring. I read, watched T.V., and talked with my fellow chemo recipients who were feeling up to talking. That's all good and fine in small doses; but it gets old very quickly day after day after day. I continued this same regimen every day through the week (with the exception of the Bleo) until I was finally done with my second round of chemo on Friday August 24th.

Like my first cycle of chemo, I felt fine during the week it was administered to me. I did however have to request some anti-nausea meds for some minor queasiness I began to feel. The drug I asked for is called Ativan; a favorite among chemo patients. If you aren't familiar with Ativan, you need to be. Ativan was a savior for me when I was receiving my chemo for two main reasons: nausea and boredom.

Ativan is a great ally in the fight against nausea. Ativan is a clear liquid that is injected to your IV line. In only a matter of minutes your body begins to relax; thus feeling no sense of tension. As only a few moments pass, you begin to feel a bit loopy as your head may begin to fall to either side, and your eyes may start to wander. Whether or not you like the feeling of being drugged, Ativan is a blessing because it will take your concentration off of the nausea to the point where you won't know you are nauseous. Usually, you will even fall asleep for an hour or two. At least, that was my experience with the drug.

Ativan is also a great ally in the fight against boredom. When you are sitting in a chair for five hours waiting for all of your drugs to drip into your veins, it is easy to get bored very quickly. Although I wouldn't admit it at the time, whenever I got bored, I would say, "Excuse me. Can I get some Ativan? I'm feeling a bit nauseous." Once I fell asleep, the next thing I knew my chemo was almost over with.

The week after my second cycle of chemo I began to feel a bit more nauseous. For the most part I was fine, but periodically I would feel uneasiness in my stomach that was strangely unfamiliar. I didn't feel like I wanted to throw-up, but I also didn't feel like eating. Despite not wanting to eat, I forced myself to because I hate the feeling of hunger pains. All and all, the week was pretty uneventful concerning nausea.

Well, There Goes The Hair

The week after my second round of chemo, my sister Tera flew up from where she lives, outside Columbus, Georgia, for the wedding of her college roommate. We all drove down together to northern Oregon where the wedding was held and checked into a beautiful hotel; Skamania Lodge. The lodge is surrounded by beautiful golf courses that look like they could challenge even Tiger Woods. I remember taking the elevator up a few floors to meet my parents in their room when a man joined me in the elevator. "Man, that course is tough I tell you!" he exclaimed, "I lost three balls today!" Laughing to myself and without missing a beat I replied, "Really? I only lost one!" I couldn't help myself. The door opened and I bid the man a good day. I burst into laughter as I walked down the hall to my parents' room. Hey, if you have to go through hell, at least have as good a time you can along the way.

It was at the lodge where I noticed my first definite physical sign that the chemo was starting to take its effect. The distance between the hotel lobby and our car was maybe 50 yards at the most, with the very slightest bit of an uphill grade. When walking from the lobby to the car, to go to the wedding, I got so exhausted that I was sweating profusely and was breathing so hard that I had to stop and take a breather. I was in pretty good shape and therefore immediately knew that something was wrong. For your sake, I won't talk about the wedding or reception since I'm sure you really couldn't care less anyway. The only thing I guess I should say is that while at the wedding, I could only go a short time standing up until I had to sit back down again. Needless to say, I didn't partake in the dancing.

The next day on our way home I was sitting in the front seat and my sister sat behind me with my mom next to her and my dad driving. "Brad? Can I touch your head for a minute?" asked Tera. "Okay" I said in a tone that suggested I wasn't sure why she wanted to. "I just want to see if you are losing hair or if it's just the way your hair is laying. She continued to poke and brush at my head until I ran my right hand through the hair on the back of my head to check for myself. Bringing my hand back into view, I found a chunk of hair pinched in-between each of my fingers. My hair had begun to fall out. Looking at my hair in disbelief I nonchalantly rolled down the window and got rid of the hair. "So, Tera. When we get home do you want to shave my head for me?" I laughed.

I didn't want to wake up every morning in a bed full of fallen out hair, so shaving my head was not a difficult decision to make at all. We got home and I went straight for my electric razor. When I came back with the razor, I found that my sister had set up a chair in the backyard, excited to start the shearing. After all my hair was gone I grabbed my trusty Mach 3 razor and shaved my head into a glossy smooth and shiny dome.

I headed out to do some errands and when I came back home I couldn't believe what I saw. I walked into the family room to see everybody staring at me smiling. It was an awkward welcoming to say the least. I then saw my dad and noticed that his once balding head was now just like mine; shaved! A huge smile came upon my face and I immediately gave him a great big hug in thanks. We were all pretty amazed as to how good he looked bald. He ended up keeping his head shaved until my hair finally began to grow back several months later. If you ask me, I think he should have kept it shaved.

Chemo Round Number 3
Doctor's Notes

Patient is now 2 weeks into his course of chemotherapy second cycle. He is feeling poorly. We would expect this really, he is neutropenic. Total white count is 1700, platelets are acceptable. He is modestly anemic with Hematocrit of 34. He has some skin toxicity, irritation of his fingertips. He also has some perirectal discomfort, although no fever. Overall, I think, fairly understandable that he feels so poorly. Suspect situation would improve shortly, as white count comes up. Cautioned him regarding fever. We will check CT scan this Thursday.

I went in once again for my biweekly check-up with Dr. Senecal. Once the blood tests came back, I found that all of the variables in my CBC had plummeted drastically and had lost about ten pounds. On a positive note, my AFP had dropped to 22.8. Things were looking good although I had begun to feel much sicker.

It was now the beginning of my third round of chemo and I began to get a bit nervous having these drugs go into my body. I had yet to feel like this. I was at a point in my treatment where I knew how my body would react to the chemo. I knew that I would feel relatively fine during the week I receive my drugs. I knew that the week after I would begin to feel more nauseous than I did in my previous round. However, I did not know how sick I would become with this next round. Would I be just a little worse; or would I be puking my guts out? What I was certain of, was that this third round would be worse than the second. At least this was going to be my final round of chemo. Whatever was going to be thrown at me I could take. Only another three weeks and this would all be over.

I went into the infusion room and sat in my usual chair tucked away in the corner. The nurses accessed my port and the drugs began to flow. It was a normal week of chemo; no different than the first two rounds. I sat for five hours a day, had a tiny bit

* * *

of an upset stomach towards the end of the week, and asked for more than my fair share of Ativan. However, there was one difference.

Doctor's Notes

The patient is starting his third course of chemotherapy. We have noted a progressive drop in the alpha-fetoprotein down to about 80 when we measured 3 weeks ago and being repeated today. His CT scan shows some reduction in the size of the tumor masses, but minimally so. My suspicion is there is residual teratoma and that we are treating the malignant component of the disease. He is doing relatively well, trying to stay positive.

I was prescribed Epogen which came in a syringe. Every day I had to inject the clear solution into the fat of my belly. Epogen is prescribed when your red blood cell count is far below normal and you are anemic. In my case my red blood cell count was at 3.92; 4.25-5.70 is considered normal. Dr. Senecal wanted to raise my red blood cell count, but most of all wanted to proactively treat the further loss of red blood cells that was certain to come. I did this myself for about four weeks and I received a shot of Aranesp (a similar drug which treats anemia) at the office once every Tuesday. I'm not the biggest fan of needles, but I had grown used to them by now. I hardly felt any pain when I gave myself the shot. The only discomfort I felt was a tiny sting in my belly, but I found that the sting was less if I warmed up the solution under my arm pit before I injected it.

Puke

It was around this time when I distinctly remember one of the first times I threw-up from my chemo. I had just left the house on the first Saturday morning after my week of chemo ended and decided to try and eat a banana for breakfast. A banana may not seem like much, but for me at that time it was a major accomplishment to be able to finish it. I was only driving for maybe five minutes when I felt the most unrecognizable sensation

Surgery Number 2 - A Change of Plan

in my stomach I had ever felt. The feeling didn't grow with time. It didn't fluctuate in intensity in any way. The feeling came without notice and stayed with me until with just seconds to spare I immediately pulled over to the side of the road and I threw-up the banana I just managed to eat. After I got the sour taste of vomit out of my mouth I stared down and saw the pile of partially digested banana spilled on the side of the road. It is a horribly upsetting feeling to see what was just a major achievement (simply eating the banana) become an immediate defeat.

Nausea did not simply make an every now and again appearance; it was booked full time. I usually threw-up about two to three times a day; and when I say "times", understand that each occurrence involves multiple heaves and purges. I know such descriptions aren't exactly pleasant or attractive, but I think it is important to describe everything I was feeling and experiencing throughout the process so you can either relate or begin to understand what I was experiencing. There is nothing quite like the feeling of what I call "chemo throw-up".

Another unforeseen symptom of the chemo was random moments of severe and often times unexplainable depression. Beginning the week my third round of chemo was administered, I noticed my emotions began to go wildly out of control. The majority of the time I was in a very positive mood, accepting and dealing with everything that fate had handed me. In-between these periods of optimism I would experience very short and brutal episodes of sadness filled with self-reflection, guilt, and tears.

These moments of sadness were sporadic. They were not triggered by upsetting topics, sights, or events. Once the tears stopped falling and the sobbing subsided I found myself questioning why I had just become so distraught. Breaking down randomly forced me accept that the chemo was starting to really take its toll on me. I knew that no matter how strong I was physically or mentally, the chemo was doing its best to break me. I refused to let it do so.

44

Surgery Number 2 - A Change of Plan

College And Cancer, A Fun Combo

When my parents and I first met with Dr. Senecal he mentioned that I would want to take a medical withdrawal from school; at the very least live at home and commute to school so I would not surround myself with the less than sterile conditions of a dorm. Be that as it may, I told him and my parents that under no circumstances would I choose to leave school or move home.

I should acknowledge that in most cases your doctor definitely knows best. However, I knew that as my treatment went on I would likely lose more and more of my freedoms as well as my dignity. I was not going to allow myself to begin losing my independence even before my treatment began. I am sure if you ask any of my family or close friends they will tell you that I am an excessively proud and stubborn person. This stand was clearly an expression of those traits.

In my first two years of college I lived on campus for only the first year; and that was only because doing so was required by the university. My second year I lived with three friends; Marisa, Britnee, and Arynn whom I mentioned earlier. Since I had lived in a house off campus the previous year, I didn't plan on living on campus again. Doing so would have felt like a step back. I knew, however, I did not want to burden a roommate(s) with my illness. I anticipated violent nausea, radical mood swings, and other side effects of chemotherapy and the cancer experience itself that would undoubtedly be bothersome. I did not want to force others to deal with my cancer as well, so I decided to move into Kreidler Hall which was a dorm of single rooms reserved for those who are of junior status or at least twenty years old. Living in Kreidler allowed me to live on campus, not trouble others with my cancer, and most importantly, it allowed me to maintain my independence.

In retrospect I realize that continuing with school and living alone had to do with more than keeping independence. I was telling myself, the world, and my cancer that I had cancer, cancer did not have me. In other words, I refused to live on

• • •

cancer's terms. I was determined to live my life as if nothing was different, as if I didn't have cancer; at least to the degree possible.

I did make one concession right off the bat, however. Toward the end of the previous semester I had registered for a full load of classes (sixteen credit hours). Although I am a very proud person, I decided to reduce my number of classes to two (six credit hours) and continue to sing with the Choir of the West as well. Cutting back on my classes would give me a fighting chance. I felt confident in my decision to be registered as a part-time student, and I would soon learn that choosing to do so was a very wise decision.

It was the first week of September and I was all moved in to Kreidler and the 2004 Fall semester just began. The first choir rehearsal of the year was about to begin so I looked at the rehearsal schedule to see in which room the Choir of the West (COW) was meeting. Lagerquist Concert Hall read the schedule. Lagerquist has got to be one of the most beautiful acoustically designed collegiate concert halls in the country, so I was happy to see that was where our first rehearsal would take place.

I made a point to arrive a bit early so I could begin placing little "gifts" on each chair for each member of the choir. A few weeks earlier I received a package from a family friend, Jodie, which contained 100 LIVESTRONG bracelets. You have more than likely seen these bright yellow bracelets worn by random people on the street to prominent politicians and celebrities. They are worn in support of those who are or who have faced cancer. (Every dollar raised by the sale of these wristbands goes toward the mission of the Lance Armstrong Foundation when purchased from their website: www.livestrong.org WARNING: Do not purchase from other sites such as eBay because the sellers are profiting rather than the cancer community.)

As the stage began to fill with my fellow singers, some looked puzzled as to why I was handing these out but most either put two and two together or they had already heard the news. On a campus of only 3,500 students, word travels pretty quickly. I had

Surgery Number 2 - A Change of Plan

arranged with the choir conductor, Kathryn Lehmann, to say a brief word at the beginning of the rehearsal.

"I am so excited to be here and to start another year of great music with wonderful people" I began. "As I am sure many of you have already heard I was diagnosed with Testicular Cancer over the summer. As you can tell from my bald head, I have already started chemotherapy and my doctors and I are confident things will turn out just fine. I've always looked at choir as a family and I am giving each of you one of these LIVESTRONG bands so if I am not able to make a performance in person, you can each wear the band to show I am there in spirit. I understand if you have any questions or concerns, so know that I am more than willing to talk about what I'm going through if you like. Thanks." The entire concert hall erupted with applause from the choir and after a few words from Professor Lehmann, the rehearsal began.

In regards to the two classes I was taking for credit, the first thing I made sure to do was to meet with the professors and fill them in on my condition. I wanted them to know that although I was feeling decent at the time, it was likely that my condition would steadily go downhill and I would do everything I could to attend class and keep up on my work. I also made arrangements with them to copy notes, get in-class handouts, etc. from fellow classmates if I was unable to attend class.

I was dreading one of my classes because I heard it was very difficult and the professor was notorious for being a harsh grader. The class was "Creating & Leading Effective Organizations" and the professor was Thom Sepic. I don't recall exactly what the project was we were to pursue and complete, but I knew that with his reputation for being a tough professor I needed to stand out somehow, so I chose to be the team leader of our four person team. On top of managing my treatment, my team consisted of one guy who was willing to work but had little if any personal drive, so he required a lot of direction. The other two were two older Korean ladies who both were ESL (English as a Second Language) students, so communication was far from easy and efficient. Needless to say, I had my work cut out for me.

* * *

Surgery Number 2 - A Change of Plan

As many of you know, living on campus can be a little bit of everything; fun, annoying, educational. But living on campus while undergoing chemotherapy is a different story. It was far from fun, and annoying doesn't even begin to describe it. I'm a firm believer that everything is educational, so I will give it that.

My room on the first floor of Kreidler Hall became to be known as "The Pharmacy" to some students in the School of Nursing because of all of the pills I had in my medicine cabinet. I remember a few instances when some nursing students visited my room so they could look at the labels and try and identify what they were for and why I was taking them.

"Warfarin" a girl said. "Why do you need thinner blood?" I then showed the port under my skin below my right collar bone and said, "It's to make sure I don't form any blood clots on my port." (An interesting side note: Warfarin originated as a rat poison designed to kill rats by making their blood so thin they would bleed out.) They went through each bottle in the cabinet and commented on each drug.

I never minded those visits. It was nice to have cheery people stop by, and I was happy to help them learn their drugs. "I'm here anyhow," I thought, "I might as well let my cancer be of good use to others." Not to mention, the girls in the PLU School of Nursing were typically pretty cute!

Of course, there were very dark times while living on campus. There were days I would wake up covered in sweat and not have enough energy to even climb out of bed. If I did have enough energy to get up, sometimes I only had enough energy to make my way to the bathroom down the hall and take a shower. Doing the simplest of tasks would sometimes take so much effort that all I could do afterwards was lay in bed and watch T.V.

When the nausea began to ramp up I learned just how much consistently vomiting can take out of you. For example, in a typical night I would be sleeping and suddenly wake up with the urgency of somebody who had blown a bull horn next to their ear, search for the garbage can I always kept next to my bed, and throw-up, trying not to get any vomit on my sheets or on myself.

Surgery Number 2 - A Change of Plan

To get the rancid acidic taste out of my mouth, I would rinse with water making sure to spit it into the garbage can rather than swallowing it. Swallowing the water that soon after throwing-up would undoubtedly cause me to throw-up immediately again. This would usually happen once to three times a night.

When it was time to wake up for the day I would be exhausted from the lack of sleep and from the purging that took place in between each temporary moment of sleep. If I determined I would be able to make it to class that day, I would shower, get dressed, and make my way to the UC (University Center) to grab something to eat. I made sure to plan extra time for eating because if I ate too quickly it would only be a matter of moments until it all came up. The weight of food hitting my stomach would guarantee another round of puking. So, I would eat slowly and only eat what I felt my stomach could handle; light things like cereal, muffins, and soft fruit. Pasta, burgers, and other such heavy foods were definitely out. As I ate I would concentrate on each swallow and react to the moment each portion of food hit my stomach. I taught myself how to flex my abs and concentrate on keeping the food down just so I wouldn't make a mess in front of all the other students there.

After finishing what little food I was able to comfortably eat I would begin to make my way to class. With my strength depleting by the day, I would walk slowly from the UC to the Admin Building only 150 yards or so away. It was common for me to stop in Red Square so I could rest and catch my breath. I would then continue on to my class.

While sitting in class I found concentrating often times difficult because my mind would drift due to all the drugs I was taking to help control my nausea and pain. Generally I was able to keep up with the discussions and note taking, but as I got further into my treatments and I took heavier doses of pain medications, concentrating became more and more difficult.

At 3:30pm I would head to MBR (the Mary Baker Russell Building) for choir rehearsal. I would often get a second wind when I got there because I was so happy to be in the presence of

● ● ●

such wonderful musicians and I loved creating beautiful vocal music. However, there were also times when I only had the energy to show up. I couldn't stand to sing. Sometimes I didn't even have the energy to sing. When that was the case, I would sit in my chair and lean against the wall as I took notes in my sheet music. At least I could take notes as a way to show my commitment to the choir.

For the days I found I just did not have the energy, I stayed in my room with the blinds closed and laid in bed while watching T.V., catching up on sleep when my body would let me. It was during one of these days when I realized just how much all the drugs were affecting me not only physically, but emotionally as well.

I was laying in bed one afternoon, too sick to go to class. I was watching the game show Family Feud and three of the five answers were revealed, but the number one and number three answers were still covered. I was certain that I knew the number one answer and as the contestants failed to call out my answer, I got more and more angry. Finally, one team got their third strike and the other team was unable to get the steal. When the last two answers were revealed, I was shocked to see my answer was not on the board. I couldn't believe my eyes! I was certain I had a right answer, but it wasn't there. My eyes then began to fill with tears and I found myself crying uncontrollably into the sheets on my bed.

Under normal circumstances this may be grounds to have somebody committed! After a few minutes of crying I wiped my eyes and as I began to realize at what I was crying, my crying turned into laughter. I couldn't believe I was being so irrational. Crying because my answer wasn't in the top five of the survey? It was just a stupid game show for crying out loud! I then gathered my emotions and told myself that I'm just letting all the drugs get the better of me. It was a slap in the face of reality, of how much impact all those drugs had on me.

I calmed down and decided to try and make myself feel a bit better by having a small snack so my hunger pains would go

Surgery Number 2 - A Change of Plan

away, or at least lessen, however temporarily. I grabbed a Costco size container of peanuts from my desk and ate two or three peanuts. As soon as I swallowed I could feel the all too familiar feeling that I was about to throw-up. I began to heave over my trusty garbage can but nothing was coming out. I could feel the partly chewed nuts climb up my throat yet unable to exit. This caused more and more heaving, but I was still not able get rid of those damned peanuts. I grabbed the water I kept next to my bed, took a huge gulp, and that was enough to piss off my stomach to throw-up that water and carry out the peanuts trapped in my throat.

In less than a minute I went from crying, to laughing, to feeling defeated by three little peanuts. I wasn't even strong enough to keep three peanuts down. I curled up in my covers and tried to fall asleep so I wouldn't have to face myself; a man who was weaker than three little peanuts.

It is funny how something so inconsequential like eating food can impact you so much that you can feel defeated by it. As I lived on campus (and throughout my entire treatment for that matter) I was forced to substitute seemingly insignificant achievements (such as getting out of bed, eating, keeping food down) for meaningful accomplishments (such as getting good grades, getting in shape, building relationships). One specific incident regarding food affected me greatly one day.

I stayed in bed one day and I felt so lazy, so useless that I convinced myself to get dressed and make my way to the UC and force myself to eat something, no matter how little it was. At a snail's pace I walked to the UC and once inside the cafeteria I settled to attempt and eat a bowl of cereal. "If I can finish this bowl of cereal" I thought to myself "today will have been a productive day." That is how much these little battles meant to me.

I grabbed a bowl of cereal, sat at a table, and began to eat. By this time I had grown used to eating slowly in the UC to not be embarrassed by those eating around me. But class was in session, so there weren't too many people around by whom I could be embarrassed. With each swallow, I concentrated on the impact it made upon my stomach, as I have learned to do to prevent from throwing-up. I managed to finish two-thirds of the bowl and I knew if I tried to eat just one more bite I would regret it. I bussed my tray and grabbed a few mini-muffins to have on hand for later in the day.

I walked out of the cafeteria and made my way through the UC to head back toward my dorm. Half way through the UC I once again felt that god-awful feeling deep in my stomach. I looked around and saw I could either make my way for the bathroom or I could try and get outside. Both were the same distance from me. I decided to try and make it outside; at least I could throw-up in a bush somewhere away from people. With a hurried walk I made my way for the doors. I knew if I ran my stomach would jostle and everything would come up right then and there.

"Thank God!" I thought to myself as I made it outside. I made a sharp left down a less used trail behind the School of Nursing. I could feel the cereal make its way up so I leaned over to the side and let it all come up on the grass next to the path. I felt as if I had taken a gut shot from Holyfield and I had just been told a loved one had died. My stomach ached and I felt completely helpless. The one thing I wanted to accomplish that day, the simple task of eating a bowl of cereal, was too much for me. I slowly made my way back to my dorm as I wiped the pooling tears in my eyes that clouded my vision. Not tears of sadness, but tears of frustration. I was not giving up, but I was beginning to ask myself how much more of this hell I could take. I crawled into bed and wiped the tears from my eyes and thought to myself, "I'll be better for this. I have cancer, cancer does not have me. I will be a better, stronger person once this is all over." and fell asleep.

I faced a similar set back the very next day. As mentioned earlier, some referred to my room as The Pharmacy because of all the pills I had to take. Most were anti-nausea pills; others were pain pills such as Vicodin. That next day, just as I finished taking my first dose of each drug, I quickly reached over and grabbed the

Surgery Number 2 - A Change of Plan

garbage can so I could once again throw-up. Sitting there in a pool of my vomit were ten clearly identifiable pills staring back at me. I sat there for a moment staring at the pills I just strove to swallow. Yet another defeat. I was so pissed off that I considered not retaking the pills. Quickly reasoning that I would only be punishing myself and not my cancer, I "bit the bullet", removed another pill from each bottle, and began the process of swallowing each of them again. Only this time, and from then on, I took each pill roughly five minutes apart. This means it took me about an hour to take my pills; a chore that should have only taken seconds.

I tell these stories realizing there is a lot of overlap and even a bit of redundancy. However, I want to stress that my life became completely different than I knew. It is important to know that what was important to me before I went through my treatment was substituted with vastly different priorities. Never did I imagine feeling a sense of accomplishment by eating a bowl of cereal or successfully taking my necessary medications. If you have cancer, I think it would be nice for you to know to anticipate this. Or, if you know of somebody who is going through treatment, you need to know that their priorities and goals will likely change. They will most likely change to something you cannot understand or appreciate. You will find that if your loved one is feeling upset because they can't manage to eat, you will be prepared to understand where they are coming from. I often found the greatest comfort talking to somebody who understood how and why I was so angry when I got so nauseous. If you are prepared, you can be that person for the one you love.

Several of the Medications I Took While Undergoing Treatment		
Medicine	Indication	Form
Darbepoetin Alfa (a.k.a. Aranesp)	Anemia (low red blood cell count)	Injection
Dexamethasone (a.k.a. Baycadron)	Nausea	Pill
Fentanyl Transdermal (a.k.a. Duragesic)	Pain	Patch
Filgrastim (a.k.a. Neupogen)	Neutropenia (low white blood cell count)	Injection
Granisetron (a.k.a. Kytril)	Nausea	IV

Hydrocodone (a.k.a. Vicodin)	Pain	Pill
Lorazepam (a.k.a. Ativan)	Pain/Sedation	Pill
Ondansetron (a.k.a. Zofran)	Nausea	Pill
Oxycodone (a.k.a. Percocet)	Pain	Pill
Potassium Chloride	Hypokalemia (low blood levels of potassium)	Pill
Prochlorperazine (a.k.a. Compazine)	Nausea	Pill

Despite all of the anger, frustrations, and personal set-backs, I did have moments of empowerment that allowed me to completely forget my illness and concentrate on having fun, like every college aged person should be able to do. Two such instances were my 21st birthday and that year's Halloween.

On September 19th, two weeks after the fall semester began, I celebrated my 21st birthday. Now, I wish I could say this traditionally momentous rite-of-passage involved the typical hard core partying, drinking to excess, and waking up in a friend's back yard with no clue how I got there or what happened the previous night. No. My birthday party was a bit more tame.

My parents arranged for my family, friends, and me to meet at Katie Downs, a staple on the Tacoma, WA waterfront known for their gourmet deep dish pizzas. My parents, my sister Andrea and her husband Mark (my other sister Tera lived in Georgia at the time), and roughly ten of my close friends met for dinner and drinks. At that time I had already completed my first round of chemo and had just started my second round.

My doctor's said I should be fine to drink a little for my birthday, but to do so in moderation. "Remember, the chemo doesn't tend to be the best for your immune system" they warned. I came to find that I didn't necessarily need their words of warning. After three drinks I began to feel a little sick, so I knew that was it for the night. If you knew me during my second year of college, you would know that three drinks were hardly getting my motor started. Three drinks was nothing!

Later that night, a group of friends and I returned to my parents' house with a 24 pack of beer and made use of the hot tub. I was only able to have one more drink, but having the opportunity to kick back, hang out with friends, and have a few drinks was the greatest thing for me because I was able to completely forget about my cancer. The night was tame, but feeling like nothing was wrong, that cancer wasn't even a part of my life, was the best birthday present I could have received. I felt happy, alive, and healthy.

The following Halloween was also a great night. By this point, my hair was long gone, as were my eyebrows, arm and leg hair, and I was much skinnier than I had been in years. My friend Marisa and her roommates planned a costume party for Halloween that I was determined to make. I shopped around for a cheap costume to wear for the night and decided on a caveman outfit, complete with arm bands and a wooden club. I am not too easily embarrassed, so I didn't care that being as tall as I am (6'5") the costume showed much more leg than intended.

By this stage in my treatment I was much more nauseous than ever before. I was two weeks out of my fourth round of chemo, and it was just one week after an emergency visit to Dr. Senecal's office (which I will talk about a little later). Regardless, it was quite the party atmosphere and I had every intention on not letting my illness get in the way of having a great time. I started with a few beers and drank each one as my friends and I watched a friend of mine, Christen, play a game of "Liquor Checkers". For those of you who aren't familiar, Liquor Checkers is your normal game of checkers played with shot glasses filled with liquor and a mixer instead of the standard black and red game pieces. One side of the board's shot glasses are filled with, say, vodka and cranberry juice. The other, maybe vodka and orange juice. This way each player knows which "pieces" are theirs. If you are jumped, you have to drink the shot(s) that was jumped. Regardless of how the game is played, somebody winds up taking all 12 shots. Needless to say, if you aren't playing very well, you can get trashed REALLY quickly.

I watched as Christen slaughtered the guy she was playing. "My turn!" I shouted. A look of horror came across her face and asked if I was sure I wanted to play. I understood her concern, but there was no way I was going to limit myself. "Damn straight!" I yelled, and I began mixing the shots.

In retrospect, I should have learned a lesson from the guy Christen trounced just before me, but, of course, I didn't. The game began and it started as most games of Checkers begin, we exchanged jumping each other for the first few moves. After that I found myself taking shot after shot after shot. "This girl is trying to kill me!" I thought to myself. A small crowd gathered around to watch the beating (maybe they were gathering to watch a guy who was clearly really sick pounding back shots).

As about half of my shot glasses were taken off the board I felt a feeling I knew all too well and dreaded. "Ugh. Not tonight. Not now" I whined. And without saying a word, I jumped out of my chair and ran to the bathroom. Marisa was close behind to make sure I was ok. With a flush of the toilet and a quick rinse of my mouth, I hugged Marisa in thanks and walked my way triumphantly back to the game. "Puke and rally!" I shouted. As the other partiers clapped, cheered, and laughed, I sat down and finished the game at which I was losing so badly. The shots I took once I rebounded managed to stay down. I built a healthy buzz and the rest of the night went without a hitch. That night I once again felt normal. I felt like I was just like everybody else there, not some sick guy to be pitied. It was awesome.

I digressed a bit chronologically to tell of two instances in which living with cancer wasn't all about pain and nausea. Let's pick up from where I began to get off track; living on campus.

As the semester was in full swing, life on campus grew more and more difficult. I had religiously been taking Vicodin to help manage the immense pain I was experiencing. Despite the large doses of Vicodin the pain persisted. To help with this pain, Dr. Senecal also prescribed two fentanyl patches which are similar to Nicoderm patches (the patches that help smokers control their cravings) in that they steadily allow the drug to absorb through the skin, thus providing a constant dose of pain managing medication. (Each patch released a dose of 50mcg per hour with a total content of 5mg. and they each measured roughly 8 inches by 8 inches.) I wore both of these on my back just below each shoulder blade. These patches allowed me to take less Vicodin and only take additional medication when the pain grew to higher than average levels. My pain was reduced substantially, but I was basically high as a kite from that point on. It was only September 27th when I started using these patches in addition to Vicodin. I had a long way to go before I would be done with all this cancer business.

Doctor's Notes

His pain control is good with patches. Nausea is obviously a lot less.

While I was on all of this pain management medication, my God-Mother Jeanine visited me on campus so we could catch-up and have lunch together. As she ate and I attempted to swallow a few bites of food, we talked about how I was feeling and how I was keeping up with school while I dealt with all that was involved with fighting my cancer. She asked me one question that took me off guard: "Do you think you will be able to keep going to classes?" I didn't know immediately what to make of such a question, because up to that point leaving school never crossed my mind.

I explained that I hadn't thought about it and that I was managing alright despite the pain, nausea, and emotional roller coasters. I was honest with her and with myself as well when I continued and said that I was simply taking everything one day at a time and if I felt that I couldn't keep up with school, or if I become too concerned about my health that I would not hesitate to move home. "I know my body is weak, but my mind is strong. I know I can keep going; at this rate that is. You know I'm not a quitter, and I don't want to give up living an independent life." I tried to explain. We talked a while longer and then we said our goodbyes.

Everything I told Jeanine was true. However, I didn't want to tell her exactly what I meant because I was afraid of how she might take it and I didn't want it to get back to my family and make them any more worried than they already were. What I really

● ● ●

meant, though, was that I was most afraid of existing and not living. I will talk more about this in the second half of the book, but I was afraid that if my life was completely void of normality, I would forget what I was fighting for. I would simply lay around the house, waiting to be cured, not knowing if that would actually happen or not. "If I am going to die I am going to die while living life" I told myself. In other words, why wait to live tomorrow if you are perfectly capable of living today?

One week after Janine visited me, I experienced one of the scariest things to happen to me since being diagnosed. Class was just dismissed and I was walking back to my dorm room so I could rest before choir rehearsal. I walked out of the doors of the Administration Building and as the throng of students rushed around me I suddenly realized that I had no idea where I was, where I was coming from, or how to get to wherever it was I wanted to go.

I knew I was in front of the Admin Building, but where was that in relation to the rest of the campus? I knew I just finished a class, but what class was it? I knew I needed to get back to my room, but where was Kreidler? I began to panic because I knew that what I was feeling was completely irrational and something I had not felt while in treatment. PLU is such a small campus! How could I get lost? Especially since I know this campus inside and out.

It was clear to me that all of the drugs I was taking were finally catching up to me. In the midst of my panic I began to cry, but I was able to bring myself together enough to not make a scene. I looked for somebody I did not know so I could ask them where Kreidler Hall was. I didn't want to ask somebody I knew because they would know immediately something was wrong with me. At least by asking somebody I didn't know they might think I was just visiting campus. I was told to walk straight and the building would be on my left. With my heart racing out of anxiety I found the dorm and managed to remember which room was mine. When I reached my room I locked the door behind me, climbed into bed, and wailed and cried into my pillows so my

• • •

neighbors or those walking by could not hear me. "What is happening to me?" I demanded to know. I couldn't come up with anything. Both physically and mentally exhausted from this horrifying event, I cried myself to sleep. I woke up an hour later with plenty of time to make my way to choir rehearsal. I didn't feel anywhere near well enough to go to rehearsal, but I knew some choir members saw me in class that day. "I don't want them to think I am not committed to COW" I told myself. So, I washed the dried tears from my face, and made my way to MBR; exhausted, frightened, and feeling sicker than ever.

The next day I decided to put what I went through the previous day behind me and see how I felt going forward. I took a day or two to do what you might call a "self-evaluation". I paid careful attention to how my nausea was progressing. Was it getting better, worse, or staying about the same? It was getting worse by the day. And my ability to concentrate; was I able to focus? Did I always know where I was on campus? Was I actually learning in my classes, or just filling a seat? There were clear gaps in my memory as to what we were learning in my classes. When I first started taking Vicodin for my pain I would take half of one pill. At this point in my treatment I was at times taking up to four whole pills to achieve the same effect, and that was in addition to the two fentanyl patches I had on my back. How could I expect to keep up with everything I demanded of myself when I resembled a zombie more than an actual person most the time?

I finally decided that since I wasn't able to learn in my classes, my nausea was getting more and more severe, and at times I had such little strength I could barely walk, it was time to leave school and move back home with my parents. It was the most difficult decision to make, yet it was so easy to do at the same time. There was no doubt in my mind that I desperately needed to move home. However, admitting that to myself was more gut retching and pride swallowing than I can describe. The major deciding factor was the scare I had not knowing where I was or what we had discussed in class. I reasoned that the little I was benefiting by continuing school did not justify the costs of paying tuition, room, and board. Lastly, I seriously began to wonder how much longer I would be able to take care of myself. Will I be able to walk to the UC for food? Might I reach a point of having such little strength that I won't be able to turn on my side to throw-up? With what seemed like thousands of questions flying around without any answers, I finally convinced myself to pick up the phone and tell my parents I needed move home.

I imagine that by know you have enough insight about me to have an idea of how difficult that call was for me to make. I am a very proud person, and making that call would confirm that I was not able to do what I set out to do; live independently. I could have wrapped up all I needed to say by saying, "Mom. Dad. I failed."

My dad answered the phone and I told him everything I was thinking and feeling. My mom quickly joined in on the conversation as well once she knew I had news to share with them both. I told them about the scare I had outside the Admin Building as well as all the questions I had about my ability to take care of myself. They loved that I wanted to move home. Finally I would be where they could keep a close eye on me and sleep a bit more soundly knowing they could help at any moment if needed. I hung up the phone feeling a huge sense of relief knowing my life would soon be much less stressful. However, I also felt an overwhelming feeling of defeat having finally given into the challenges my treatment had forced me to face.

The next day I scheduled meetings with my three professors (my two business professors and the director of COW, Professor Lehmann) to let them know that I was taking a medical withdrawal from the semester. I first met with Professor Sepic, the professor of my Creating & Leading Effective Organizations class, and the words he had for me meant more than he could have known. "I'm not surprised," he said, "but I am saddened that this had to happen. You have done a wonderful job leading your team. I know you had quite a few challenges with your team (he was referring to my three "less than ideal" team members) but you led them well. I don't think they stand much of a chance without you."

This was coming from a professor who had the reputation of being notoriously difficult to please and despite everything I was facing, I was evidently doing a great job as Team Leader. "I was looking forward to giving at least one 'A' this semester" he said jokingly. I thanked him for his kind words and for being a great teacher as well. He asked me to keep him updated on my status then we shook hands and I went off to go talk with Professor Lehmann.

When I went into Professor Lehmann's office I had the suspicion that she knew what I was going to say. Regardless, I told her that I decided to leave school for the semester. As she had been since she first learned of my cancer, she was very supportive and said she agreed with my decision. "Although I won't be taking classes any longer for the semester, may I still continue with the choir?" I asked. As I said before, COW is like a family and I did not want to leave them one bass short. Also, I am a firm believer in the healing power of music. Every day in rehearsal, no matter how horrible I was feeling, I always felt slightly better as I sang and listened to the beautiful chords fill the room. It was as if the music itself reached deep inside of me and pulled out the pain I was feeling. Professor Lehmann said I was more than welcome to stay with the choir and to come to rehearsals as I felt up to it. I was relieved to hear I would be able to have at least one normal aspect of my life intact.

The day I moved back home I found my dad had moved my bed from my room upstairs down to the first floor in his den/office. He knew that if I was feeling bad enough to make myself move home I must be feeling pretty awful. He foresaw that I would likely continue to lose strength and that it might even become too much of a chore to climb the stairs. So, from day one I lived out of my dad's den. It was nice to know that if things did get that bad, I had the assurance of a bed on the first floor available.

● ● ●

61

Surgery Number 2 - A Change of Plan

Doctor's Notes

(From Doctor Frank Senecal to Pacific Lutheran University)
RE: To Whom It May Concern:

Brad Lubken is a patient under my care for a serious medical condition. As you may be aware, he has required very intensive therapy over the past several months. He is improving. The therapy itself however is very debilitating, and Brad has found it extremely difficult to keep up in his studies.

It is with real regret that he feels he is not able adequately keep up with his studies at this point, and we are asking that you and the University consider his present status and permit him to withdrawal without hopefully any penalty.

Brad is, as you know, a very motivated, young man. It is his serious desire to return to school quickly upon his recovery, and we think that will be possible in the course of events.

If I can provide any additional information I would be happy to do so.

Sincerely,

Frank M. Senecal, M.D./kp

Nearly every Monday through Thursday I would take the ten mile drive from my parent's house to PLU for rehearsal. I made every effort to make it first of all because I was committed to the choir. Also, I just wanted to get out of the house so I could feel as if I had accomplished something each day. "Cabin Fever", as they call it, can be extremely demoralizing, and I didn't need that on my mind on top of everything else.

The 2004 Fall Choral Concert was finally here! I looked forward to the concert every year because it was the first formal performance of the concert season and it allowed the choirs of PLU to showcase how far they had come in just six short weeks, and it gave a glimpse of what was to come later on in the year. I had made the majority of the rehearsals since leaving school and I was well prepared on the repertoire. In my mind nothing would prevent me from singing in these two concerts (one on Tuesday and one on Thursday).

The week before the concert, I told Professor Lehmann I had every intention of performing, but that it was possible I could be really sick those nights. We would have to play it be ear. For the first concert, I decided although I was feeling pretty sick and weak, I was up to singing (yet another display of my stubbornness). I showed up to Lagerquist (the concert hall on campus) in my tuxedo ready to sing. I was so excited to be participating that there were times I even forgot I was sick.

The concert began with other choirs performing first, leading up to the Choir of the West. Moments before we were to process on stage I began to feel very tired and weak. I knew that I would not have the stamina to stay standing for the whole set. Getting light-headed I could barely stay standing backstage. Just before the doors were to open for us to enter the hall, Professor Lehmann had a stagehand place a tall stool where I would soon be standing. This was a life saver! The choir then began to process onto the stage and I took my place on the stool as if it was all planned in advance. Professor Lehmann rose her hands, winked at me as if to say, "Don't worry, I'm looking out for you", and we began our set.

Our performance was exquisite and well received. After our bows at the end of our performance we recessed off the stage and when I reached backstage I wiped a tear of sheer happiness off my cheek. It didn't take me long to realize that this was the first

• • •

happy tear I shed throughout my treatment. I felt more empowered than any book could ever begin to try and explain.

Our Plan Just Changed (Chemo Round Number 4)

When I began my third round of chemo on Monday September 20th, I was so excited because it was going to be my final round. I did not like feeling sick. I did not like not eating. I did not like the idea that I had living cancer in my body. I was excited for my biweekly check-up with Dr. Senecal because I knew that my AFP level would have dropped below six (the normal level for a healthy person) as expected. Unfortunately, my expectations didn't turn out as planned.

The week after I completed my third round of chemo, I went into the exam room and sat in a chair to wait for Dr. Senecal to come in just like I had in all my previous visits. A few minutes had passed when Dr. Senecal entered the room. I stood up to shake his hand and he asked how I had been feeling since my latest round of chemo. We stood and talked about my drastic increase in nausea and how I was coping with it all. "Well," he said, "let's take a seat and discuss your latest blood test results." I thought he was going to congratulate me on a fight well fought and that my treatment was finally over.

I was not expecting to hear what Dr. Senecal was about to say. "Your recent AFP level dropped as expected; but, it didn't drop as much as we had hoped. You see, you know we are aiming for an AFP level at six or below, and this last round of chemo has left you with an AFP count of 13.5. I'm very concerned about this because this means there are cancer cells that are still living. They are fighting the chemo. I'm afraid we'll have to give you a fourth round of chemo to kill these remaining cells. I have to be perfectly honest at a time like this. Only 10% of Testicular Cancer patients have resistant cells after their third round of chemo. And, only about 50% of that 10% are cured."

It took me a minute to let that bit of info sink in. In my head it sounded like I was only given a 50% chance of living. In my head, it was a coin flip as to whether I would die or not. He

• • •

then continued, "Also, I have been corresponding with another doctor throughout your treatment about you and I would like you to see him at the completion of this fourth round of chemotherapy. This is a very rare cancer where most oncologists might see a case like this maybe once every few years, he sees this type of Testicular Cancer every day. I'd like him to decide if you will be an acceptable candidate for surgery at that time, and if so Dr. Vaccaro can proceed with the operation. This doctor's name is Dr. Craig Nichols. He's a great doctor. In fact, he was one of Lance Armstrong's oncologists."

Doctor's Notes

(From Dr. Frank Senecal to Dr. John Vaccaro)

Dear John:

Brad is going to receive his fourth cycle of chemotherapy for moderate risk testicular cancer starting next week. As you know, he has residual disease that I am sure will remain present after he completes the chemotherapy. His alpha fetoprotein had dropped to a normal range but residual masses exist and are somewhat cystic in character, both at the aortocaval area and the right pelvic area.

I suspect that you might well want to proceed with surgery three or four weeks after he completes his chemotherapy.

I will keep you posted from my perspective.

Sincerely,

Frank M. Senecal, M.D./kp

* * *

Surgery Number 2 - A Change of Plan

It was Monday October 11th and time for me to receive my unprecedented fourth round of chemo. The week prior I had my AFP checked again and it had dropped to 11.1, still too high. I walked in to the office tired, skinny, and nauseous. Although I regained most of the weight I lost in my second round, I had lost over twenty pounds during my latest chemo cycle. I knew this last round was going to be the Mount Everest of chemo rounds. I knew it would not be easy by any means because it was the first time I showed up to chemo already feeling sick. That had never happened before. I had always shown up feeling relatively fine and began to get sick a week later.

Every day I asked for Ativan. I didn't just ask, I begged. The feeling of nausea was so prevalent that I reasoned in my head that when (not if) I vomit, I would prefer to be asleep when it happened. I didn't care if it got all over me and I was so sick that I didn't care if I choked on all that yummy stuff coming up. I had simply had my fill of throwing up for one lifetime and refused to taste the acidity and feel that unsettledness in my stomach again. I wasn't giving up, I simply refused to work with cancer any longer.

Throughout the week, I ate on and off. I usually didn't feel like eating due to my nausea, but I forced myself to eat little amounts each day to maintain at least some weight. I also had a second motive for keeping my weight up though. I had planned in advance that I would not eat during the week after getting this fourth round of chemo because of my utter hatred for vomiting. "If I don't eat I can't throw up." It made logical sense to me. Sure, it wasn't a healthy thing to do, but I didn't care. Like I said, I refused to live on cancer's terms any longer. I was calling the shots now.

So, This Is What Death Feels Like

Once the week after my fourth round of chemo was upon me, I kept to my "starvation" diet. I had no will to eat because keeping an empty stomach eased my nausea. The first two days of not eating (or drinking for that matter) hurt like hell. But, I was fairly comfortable the rest of the week. My body must have

● ● ●

accepted my hunger and blocked the thought of eating from my mind. Nevertheless, I continued to feel more nauseous than I ever thought I could be in my entire life. I didn't have anything in my stomach to throw up, but that didn't keep my body from constantly heaving over and over and over again. My body knew I had more poison in it than ever and it wanted to get rid of it by any means necessary.

Consuming no food or liquids for an entire week does not come without severe consequences. I was already becoming anemic from the chemo, and not drinking any water made my condition even worse by becoming extremely dehydrated. You'll recall that I had lost significant weight during my other rounds of chemo. I was losing weight then when I was eating. Not eating at all resulted in an unforeseeable drastic loss of forty pounds in just one week. My eyes were sunk. My face was boney. I was weak. I was not myself.

That next weekend (once the fourth round was over) I noticed I felt funny when I stood up after lying on the couch. I'm sure you are familiar with the dizziness and lightheadedness you might feel from time to time when you stand up too quick; however, every time I stood up I would experience such a feeling; only much, much worse. When I stood up, the room would spin, my vision would blur, I would see only in black and white, and I would momentarily black-out, collapsing to the floor. I was confined to my house because I had to crawl everywhere I went. If I tried walking around the house I had to carry my king sized down comforter with me to cushion my fall that was certain to follow. My entire left side was bruised from falling over and over again.

Why was such a frightening symptom occurring? To begin with, as I mentioned before, my red blood cell count had been drastically lowered due to my chemotherapy. In fact, my red blood cell count was down to 1/4 the amount of a normal, healthy person. To give you an idea of how anemic I was, the lack of red blood cells (and therefore a lack of oxygen in my blood) resulted in never-ending splitting headaches. I had an MRI on my head to rule out the possibility of a brain tumor causing the pain. Thankfully

* * *

that scan tested negative for brain cancer. Secondly, I was radically dehydrated since I refused to drink anything. I was so dehydrated that when I pinched the skin on the back of my hand, the skin sank down at the speed of warmed molasses. Also, my blood pressure was below normal making it difficult for my heart to pump the optimal amount of blood to my brain.

Dehydration alone could have been reason enough for the adverse effects of my diet; but the combination of a low red blood cell count, dehydration, and extreme weight loss contributed to my inability to walk. When I stood up my blood pressure dropped even further than what it already was, thus allowing even less blood up to my brain. The reduced amount of blood traveling to my brain had less oxygen in it than it should have because of my anemia (the purpose of red blood cells is to carry oxygen). The lack of oxygen reaching my brain caused me to pass out.

I was not scheduled to return to my doctor's office, but I had deteriorated so much over the weekend that on Monday my dad drove me to Dr. Senecal's office as my grave condition was a concern to all of us. Just getting into the large Ford F-150 truck was tough enough of a challenge. I collapsed twice on my way to our garage, and my dad had to help me walk to the truck and climb in. I barely had enough strength to keep my head up as we were driving to the doctor's office.

Once at the office, we parked the truck and I waited for my dad to help me out of the truck and into the building. At a snail's pace, we walked towards the building; every few steps taking a break due to exhaustion. I believe I fell once or twice into my dad's arms on our way to the building. Once inside the hallway leading to the elevator, I had my dad walk on one side of me with the wall on the other for support. Finally, after just a few steps, I got dizzy and passed-out once again. This time I was not able to stand back up. I laid there for a while with my dad when a lady walked by shocked at the sight she saw in front of her. "Would you like me to get him a wheel chair?" she asked my dad as she already began to retrieve one. My dad lifted me into the wheel chair and wheeled me into Dr. Senecal's office.

● ● ●

Surgery Number 2 - A Change of Plan

Doctor's Notes

The patient is very nauseated today. Although, his peripheral counts are acceptable, he is clearly quite dehydrated having kept good in the past couple of days. We are going to care for him in the outpatient area today with IV hydration.

As my dad checked me in to the office, I experienced yet another pain I had never felt before. It wasn't a pain of physical anguish; rather, an emotional pain of knowing that there is something seriously wrong happening to me. It wasn't the same pain as when I found I had cancer because this time I could actually feel and witness the physical symptoms of something being wrong. I knew what I was feeling was not normal and could not be healthy, so I was scared out of my mind, wondering if I would be ok. "Am I dying? I wouldn't be surprised if this is what one may feel like on their way toward the white light."

The nursing staff was ordered to give me saline mixed with Potassium. I was wheeled into a more private room where I spent approximately six hours a day for three days. I was in a state of numbness where I was sad, but not sad; scared, but not scared. I wanted to cry, but I wasn't able to work up the energy to wrinkle my face and breathe hard. Instead, tears began to fall down my face without any of the usual energy consuming reactions that accompany crying. The tears pooled in my eyes and I had to turn my head to the side to let them fall away.

Doctor's Notes

The patient received chemotherapy last week and clearly is feeling weak and very tired. His energy level is low. He had a difficult weekend. We are planning on giving hydration over the next 3 days, and we will send him home with that as well. We will recheck alpha-fetoprotein today and CBC. Because of past neutropenia, we will proceed with Neulasta.

* * *

Surgery Number 2 - A Change of Plan

Toward the end of the week I began to feel much better. I was finally able to stand up without falling by that same Friday. That week I had my usual check-up after having a round of chemo and I found that my AFP count was at 7.4; just barely above normal. I also found that my red blood cell count was steadily rising and now at 3.73; just 12% below normal. It looked like I was not dying after all.

Doctor's Notes

The patient is a young man that we are treating for a carcinoma of the testis. This appeared to be a mixed germ cell tumor with both teratoma and embryonal components. Alpha-fetoprotein was the major marker that was elevated, although LDH was modestly elevated. Preoperatively, his LDH was above 2000, postoperatively just prior to chemotherapy on August 11, 2004 his alpha-fetoprotein was approximately 800. We have seen a progressive drop in the alpha-fetoprotein, but it clearly has leveled off in terms of rate of decline. As I marked out the half-lives of the marker, I would estimate that he should have reached a normal level after about 8 weeks. That's later than what was seen in Brad's case. Last measurement was 11, just after his fourth cycle, will be re-checked today. I imagine that it will be down to a normal level, however, I am not convinced to that and would favor restaging the disease completely and further discussions with Dr. Vaccaro. Because of my considering regarding the alpha-fetoprotein, I would also like to discuss with Dr. Nichols at Oregon Health Sciences University. I know Dr. Nichols from the past and his reputation on testicular cancer. As I e-mailed him, he was receptive to the idea of seeing the patient. That might well mean that he would undergo surgical resection there as well.

Making Good Use Of My Cancer

I drove myself to Curtis High School, my Alma Matter, and walked to the class room of Mrs. Jacobson, my health teacher

● ● ●

when I went to school there. The school day had just ended so I was making my way through throngs of students anxious to go home. I entered Mrs. Jacobson's classroom and before I could say hello, she looked at me and said, "Hat please!"

Clearly, she thought I was a student and she did not appreciate a student wearing a hat in her classroom. I complied and removed the black Guinness beanie that was protecting my bald head from the cool fall air. She finished talking to her students and then turned to me. Noticing my hairless scalp, the smiling expression on her face fell away she said, "Oh crap. You have cancer, don't you?" I could just see her saying to herself, "Insert foot in mouth."

Laughing I said, "Sure enough!" She then realized who I was; not a student, but a former student who had come upon tough times. We sat and talked for a while discussing what I was experiencing, how I was feeling, and what the future looked like. My intent was to ask her if there was an opportunity to speak to her classes sometime during the year to tell them my story and inform them not just about cancer, but how cancer can happen at a young age. Before I could request a speaking opportunity she asked if I would be willing to do so. "Whenever you want to come in you are welcome to. I'll just adjust the class agenda accordingly" she said. We penciled in some days for me to speak, realizing that my ability to come depended on how I felt that day. Leaving the class room I was so excited to have gotten the opportunity to tell my story to others. I would finally be able to make some good out of this horrible disease.

The day before I was supposed to make my first appearance at one of Mrs. Jacobson's classes was when I had the emergency visit to Dr. Senecal's. I called to regretfully let her know I had to postpone my talk. Of course, she understood completely and we rescheduled for another day the next week.

I felt much better that next week and was able to speak to some of her classes as planned. As Mrs. Jacobson introduced me, I had flashbacks to when I was in high school and visitors came to speak. It was great because it was a change of pace from the

* * *

typical class. But, it was also dreadful because the speaker was usually so boring it was all you could do to keep your eyes open. I made a point not to be like those speakers I remembered.

I told my story, but I did so with jokes and with what energy I could pull together. Regardless of how difficult things may be (regardless of the challenge), you need to keep a sense of humor about it; especially when it comes to something like cancer. For example, I like to say that the worst thing about Testicular Cancer is that I now walk in large circles to the left because I am left heavy! This can be a very uncomfortable topic for many people, so I find that making light of it at times allows others to be receptive to learning about it.

Toward the end of the first class, I opened the floor for any questions the students had. This was a fairly enlightening time for me. One question I got was, "What exactly is cancer?" I realized that not only had I never been asked that question before, but I never really thought about it myself. Some people giggled at the question, but affirmed that it was a really good question. "We hear about cancer all the time, but I don't think many people truly know what it is" I said. "When people hear 'cancer', people tend to think of words like bald, sick, and death. But they don't really know what it is."

"Basically, cancer is when one rogue cell in your body gets pissed off, changes slightly, and grows more and more cells like it" I explained. Sure, it may not be the most clinical definition of cancer, but in its essence, that is what cancer is. Regardless of the group to which I am speaking, this is usually how I like to describe cancer. People tend to go deaf when they hear medical mumbo jumbo.

As would be expected, the next question was, "What can piss off a cell?" Laughing because of the candidness of the conversation, and because I was excited to see the students were really engaged, I explained that many things can anger a cell. "Tobacco and alcohol can cause cancer in the lungs and liver. Radiation caused a lot of different cancers in people around Hiroshima, Nagasaki, and Chernobyl. Chemicals in everyday

● ● ●

products can even cause cancer." I noticed a lot of eyebrows go up when I said that, so I asked, "Did you know shampoo and toothpaste contain chemicals that can cause cancer?" I went on to say that they should continue to brush their teeth and wash their hair, but many of the chemicals in products we use every day contain carcinogens.

One of my favorite questions I got from a student went something like this in a very nervous voice: "When you had your first surgery... Did you, um... I mean were you allowed to, uh... You know... Did they..." I figured I'd help him out and I said, "Do you mean, was I allowed to keep my removed testicle?" The class (Mrs. Jacobson included) burst out laughing and the kid exclaimed, "Yes!"

"You must have seen the movie Tomcats," I laughed. In this movie there is a funny (and completely impractical) scene where a guy with testicular cancer asks his friend to get his testicle back for him as a souvenir. His friend tries to get it for him, but the testicle bounces all around the hospital, eluding the friend. I tried to keep somewhat of a straight face as I explained that you cannot keep something like that; that it is medical waste.

All of these questions are exactly why I wanted to speak about cancer. It is important to clarify the misunderstandings that abound as well as educate others so they know what to look for in themselves. Perhaps most importantly, I think it is important for young people (say, those under 50) to hear my story so they can acknowledge that cancer is in fact possible at a young age. I like to think that if one of these kids feels something unfamiliar, instead of assuming it is nothing, they will remember I spoke to them when they were in high school, and that will prompt them to see a doctor.

I also enjoy speaking because it gives them insight to the mind of somebody who has gone through treatment. I am convinced that we have all been affected by cancer in some manner. If you know somebody undergoing treatment, how should you talk to them? I hope my speaking efforts (and this book for that matter) will teach people that although every person is different, I have never met a survivor who wants a pity party thrown for them. I believe an educated person is less likely to inadvertently speak like that to somebody facing cancer.

I was scheduled to speak to more of Mrs. Jacobson's classes the next week; however, effects of my fourth round of chemo hit me once again. Since I felt like I was close to death, I rescheduled. When I was finally able to speak to the remainder of the classes, I learned more about myself, my experience, and the value of telling my story.

Besides speaking at Curtis, I have spoken at my college campus (Pacific Lutheran University) and various community meetings. At PLU, I spoke at a leadership conference where I spoke to a small group of people about my cancer experience and how I have become a better person because of it. I was invited to speak at a local Rotary Club meeting after two members read my bio in the program for a performance at PLU in which I sang. Also, a family friend and fellow survivor (who has sadly since passed) invited me to speak at a planning committee meeting for the Tacoma, Washington Relay For Life.

At each of these speaking opportunities I have been overwhelmed reception I have received. I have gotten standing ovations, people have waited to shake my hand or give me a hug, and they have confided in me with their own stories about their bouts with cancer or those of their loved ones. It did not take me long to realize that my speaking, for one reason or another, is inspirational to those who listen. This is great to hear because I have often doubted the value of my story.

Why is my story any better than anybody else's? Why would people want to spend their time listening to me? Aren't I too young to offer anything worthwhile? These and countless other questions have raced through my mind at one time or another. However, I now realize that although my story is not necessarily "better" than anybody else's, I am willing to share it with the world while others are less willing to do so. I have found that people find comfort and trust in others who can relate to them when it is often hard to find such people. It is for that reason that

• • •

Surgery Number 2 - A Change of Plan

I continue to seek out speaking opportunities and why I am writing this book. I have said it before and I will say it again... the cancer community is more than a general group of people. It is a family. And I am more than willing to commit a large part of my heart and my life to my family.

5. Referral For Surgery – Retroperitoneal Node Dissection Complete

Sharing Lance Armstrong's Oncologist
Doctor's Notes

(From Dr. Frank Senecal to Dr. Craig Nichols)

Dear Doctor Nichols:

I have asked Brad to see you regarding his diagnosis of a mixed germ cell tumor with mature teratoma and embryonal call components.

Brad presented with a painless testicular mass in the beginning of August of 2004. He underwent a radical orchiectomy by Doctor Vaccaro, one of our urologists in the Tacoma area. CT scans demonstrated a retroperitoneal mass on the right side, as well as an upper pelvic mass that looked more cystic in structure.

His pre-operative alpha-fetoprotein was in the area of 2000. His post-operative alpha-fetoprotein was approximately 1000 (802 on 08-09-04, the first day of chemotherapy). His HCG has been normal.

The patient had a PET scan pre chemotherapy that demonstrated the lesions in the upper right pelvis and retroperitoneum, but no other masses. CT scan of the abdomen, pelvis, and chest were performed as well. There is no evidence of chest disease.

Brad received chemotherapy in the form of V-16, Cisplatinum, and Bleomycin at standard doses. He tolerated this therapy well during the first two cycles but had more nausea during the subsequent

• • •

two cycles. I elected to give four courses of chemotherapy because the degree of elevation of the alpha-fetoprotein at the time of diagnosis, putting him in an intermediate risk group.

His alpha-fetoprotein fell precipitously during the first two courses, but then I recognized after cycle three that there appeared to be a plateau occurring. However, after the fourth cycle of chemotherapy, one week after completion, his alpha-fetoprotein has dropped to a normal level of 6.4.

He is in the process of recovering from his therapy.

He has required Neupogen to support the neutrophil count with his chemotherapy as well as Aranesp.

CT scan and PET scans are pending and should accompany him to his visit with you.

Both Doctor Vaccaro and I are concerned regarding the marker and what appears to be a plateau, even though it is at a normal level at this point.

The patient may well be a candidate for proceeding to retroperitoneal node dissection in the near future, but obviously the issues of persistent malignancy are raised.

I should mention that I held the last two weeks of Bleomycin with cycle four because of the indication for surgery.

I appreciate your help very much in Brad's case. Thanks for assessing him. Certainly if additional chemotherapy were indicated I would be happy to

Referral For Surgery – Retroperitoneal Node Dissection Complete

facilitate here in Tacoma. If it is felt he should proceed to surgery I have indicated to the family that you have conveyed to me that your urological surgeons are quite facile with the nerve sparing procedure, and I think the family would be comfortable with proceeding with surgery in Portland.

Sincerely,

Frank M. Senecal, M.D./kp

My mom, dad, and I drove from Tacoma, Washington to Portland, Oregon. After three hours of driving we reached Oregon Health Sciences University (OHSU) where we were to meet with Dr. Craig Nichols. After checking in, we sat in the waiting room for several minutes waiting to be escorted back to the examination room where we would finally meet with the "world famous" Dr. Nichols. As I sat in the room with my parents, I could not help but think "Wow! Lance Armstrong was in this exact same office!" I usually don't get star struck, but since I knew what Lance had been through and I could relate so well to his ordeal, I was awed simply to be in the same examination room he had probably once been in.

After my vitals were taken, an overall average man (average height, weight, etc.) entered the room and introduced himself as Dr. Nichols. He had no extraordinary features about him, but one thing did grab my attention and that was when he entered the room we couldn't help but feel to be in the presence of an exceptionally knowledgeable doctor and we were therefore very comforted; even though he didn't smile much. He had a presence about him that exemplified knowledge and capability. I suppose one could mistake his demeanor for arrogance, but we viewed it more like confidence.

We talked for a few minutes and I answered the questions he asked. He finally acknowledged that he and Dr. Senecal had

* * *

been corresponding about my case since I was diagnosed. And then the moment of truth came upon us as Dr. Nichols began to say, "So, as you know I've been reviewing your lab results to determine if you are okay or not to head into surgery. Your AFP counts have dropped very quickly when you began your chemo, but towards the end, the numbers started to plateau. Your most recent AFP count taken October 25th was just above normal at 6.4." He was basically restating everything we already knew. "Even so, I am very confident that although your numbers do suggest there are still a few living cancerous cells in your body, our world class surgeons can successfully extract both of the tumors as well as any resistant cells. I think we can go ahead and schedule your surgery." My parents and I were relieved that Dr. Nichols felt comfortable about going into surgery. We never imagined we would ever be excited for surgery, but this meant cancer would finally be out of my body.

As we left the examination room Dr. Nichols said if we had time he would like us to meet with the surgeon that would be performing my surgery; Dr. Mitchell H. Sokoloff. There was no way I was going to pass up the opportunity to meet the man who was going to saw open my body, so we made an appointment for three hours later; once Dr. Sokoloff was out of surgery. Because we didn't want to by chance miss Dr. Sokoloff's availability, we waited in his waiting room for the three hours he was in surgery instead of leaving and coming back.

Meeting The Man Who Would Save My Life

After the very long wait, we were finally escorted into yet another examination room. A fairly young doctor came in and introduced himself as Dr. Sokoloff. I was immediately impressed by him because, unlike most other surgeons I had known, he actually had good patient-doctor demeanor. Dr. Sokoloff is the exception, but I still have it set in my mind that those who become surgeons do so only because the people they have to deal with are always under anesthesia. In my experience my surgeons have always been very book smart but not exactly "social creatures".

Referral For Surgery – Retroperitoneal Node Dissection
Complete

Once we first met Dr. Sokoloff, any tensions we had about the upcoming surgery were quickly eased. When he entered the room, it looked as if he was excited to meet us. With an energetic presence and a big smile, he introduced himself to my parents and me. "Hello Brad," he said, "I've heard a lot about your case." He then began to describe the placement and size of the two tumors in my abdomen and my right hip, and he must have sensed some confusion on our part because before he continued talking he said, "Have you seen your films yet?"

"No," I replied.

"Well then, come on back and I'll show you exactly what's going on inside."

We walked up to one of those light boards that are used to look at medical films and he put up two sheets of my CT scan up for us to see. "Now you see here?" he asked pointing to one of the pictures, "This looks normal; but, in the next picture we begin to see some white appear just above the top of your right leg, in your hip. In the next picture it gets larger. And, again, in the next picture more white appears. Over here we see even more white. This white next to your pelvis is the tumor in your right lower hip." He placed his hand on my lower abdomen so I knew exactly where the tumor was.

We then looked at my abdominal CT scan to find my second tumor. Like the first time, we went frame by frame to follow the progressive size of the tumor. "This one (the second tumor) is in your left abdomen, connected to your Vena Cava and Aorta from your heart" he stated as he placed his hand just below and to the left of my sternum. I knew that I had a tumor in that general region, but neither I nor my parents had any idea that it was connected to the two largest arteries leading to and from the heart! I looked over to my parents and gave a nervous laugh as I noticed a look of relative terror on their faces.

"But aren't these in my back?" I asked. Through the research I had done, I learned that testicular cancer usually begins to spread via the lymph nodes and that the lymph nodes are on the lining of your back. Plus, Dr. Senecal had told me long before that both tumors were connected to the lymph nodes.

"Yes, they are" he replied. Touching my back where the tumors were, he explained, "The tumors are actually here and here" pointing to my right lower back and mid-way up the left side of my back. "They are growing from the lymph nodes, but also growing outwards" moving his hands to my abdomen.

Now having been educated as to where my tumors were, we went back to the examination room and got down to business. He then began to describe the process of the surgery; the prep, the actual surgery, and the recovery. He literally grabbed a pen and paper and began to draw out the surgery, step-by-step, in front of us.

Now that we knew what to expect, there was only one thing to do before heading into surgery. Dr. Sokoloff asked that I have one unit of blood on hand at the surgery just in case it was needed. Sure, there was other blood that could have been used, but since I had perfectly healthy blood he preferred I used my own instead of using the limited supply of blood available from donors. We left Dr. Sokoloff's office much more at ease than we anticipated. Dr. Sokoloff spent so much time with us (over an hour) detailing the surgery that we didn't even have any questions for him at the end. We headed for the car to return home without any worry of the surgery to come because we knew I would be in the best of hands. The only better hands to be in would be in those of God Himself.

Donating Blood To Myself... That's Different!

I found that the closest place I could deposit and have my blood shipped to OHSU for surgery for free was in Longview, Washington; a good 90 miles away from my house. I got on the phone and called the blood bank with which I had donated many times before (Cascade Blood Services) and asked if I could deposit my blood there since it was close to my house. I found that I was allowed to deposit my blood there, but for them to ship it to the hospital they would charge me $150. So, I decided to drive the 90 miles to Longview rather than pay the $150. Why not? It would be good for me to get out.

Having blood drawn from your arm is the same process whether it is to donate, or to have on hand for surgery. Before I had cancer I had already donated one gallon and one pint of blood (nine donations) so I knew the process of donating pretty well. First, you are asked to lie on a table and pick an arm from which to donate. Sometimes you may not have a choice if one arm has a vein that is difficult to find. Next, iodine is rubbed onto the skin with a cotton swab, which looks like a giant Q-tip, where the needle will be inserted, to sterilize the area. You are then given something soft to squeeze for a moment or two to swell the vein and the nurse will ask you to stop squeezing as she gently inserts the needle. I know most people don't like the thought of needles, but believe me when I say that the size of the needle they use to take blood is small enough that it doesn't hurt too badly; especially if you've been undergoing chemo with the constant needle pricks. Once the needle is in, a piece of tape secures it in place. From there on you simply lay back and resume squeezing until the nurse says you have donated your one pint of blood and you are done. To keep your arm from bleeding, a bandage is placed over the access site and you are free to go on your way (after eating some free cookies and drink some juice, of course).

Before I was allowed to deposit my blood and schedule my surgery, I had to get my red blood cell count back up to an acceptable level. Weekly I would continue to receive my shot of Aranesp to get my red blood cell count above that mark. Finally, after a few weeks of injections, my red blood cell count was back to normal and I was allowed to deposit my blood. I drove down to Portland and did my thing. When I got to the Red Cross building, I can't say I was too impressed by its cleanliness. The building was old and smelled like it too. There was garbage on the ground in places, boxes all over the place, and the carpet was frayed and dirty. I was there for maybe fifteen minutes and was back on the road to drive the 90 miles back home.

* * *

Referral For Surgery – Retroperitoneal Node Dissection
Complete

Surgery Number 3: The Big One

It was nearing the moment of truth. The day before my surgery my dad picked-up a prescription for me which was meant to "flush me out", if you know what I mean. He brought home two glass bottles of cherry flavored magnesium citrate. I heard the taste was bad enough to make you gag, but I wasn't too concerned about that. I felt that if I could go through what I already had, I could go through pretty much anything. Besides, I've gotten used to the Barium contrast shakes I had to drink prior to each CAT scan. What I was not especially looking forward to was paying the bathroom a visit every half hour or so.

Not eating anything 24 hours prior to surgery, I took my first sip and was glad to find that it didn't taste all that bad. I was able to finish the first bottle with relatively little trouble. But, towards the bottom of that bottle the overwhelmingly sweet taste of cherry began to make me feel sick to my stomach. Each additional sip began to taste increasingly more like pure cherry syrup. Grimacing, I finished the second bottle right before the stuff began to kick in.

Sitting on the couch in our family room, I felt a grumbling in my gut and knew the fun was about to begin. I stood quickly and got to the bathroom, did what I had to do, and came back to the couch to watch TV. Since I had just gone to the bathroom, I didn't expect for nature to call immediately; but to my surprise, after only five minutes or so I had to rush back to the bathroom again. I had been racing back and forth to the bathroom for two hours when my mom, dad, sister, and I piled into the car to drive down to Portland, Oregon for my surgery in the morning. Right off the bat, once we hit the road, I had to ask my dad to find a restroom. Once again I did my business and went on my way. After a mile or more down the road nature called again! This was getting ridiculous! We joked that it was going to be like this the entire drive down to Portland and it would take all night just to get there. But, the porcelain gods finally gave me a break and my

• • •

digestive system began to calm down. All and all, I guess you can say I had a pretty "shitty" ride.

Early the next morning my dad and I woke up so we could get to OHSU in time to complete all the monotonous paperwork and pre-surgical stuff. We planned for my mom and sister to wake up later and meet the two of us just before I went into surgery so they could sleep in, yet still offer a few words of encouragement. However, while we were taking care of the pre-surgical necessities a nurse approached us and said that (for one reason or another) the surgical team would like to move up my surgery time from 9:00am to 7:00am; it was 6:30am when I was told this.

Although I would have liked to have seen my mom and sister before my surgery, and I knew they wanted to see me before I went into surgery as well, I was rushed to finish prepping for surgery. As I was doing so, the same nurse as before came in once again and said Dr. Sokoloff wanted me to have an epidural to help with the post-surgical pain. To be perfectly honest, up until then I had no idea what an epidural was. I associated the word epidural with women giving birth. I figured an epidural was just an IV drip of pain medication; I didn't know an epidural was basically a needle shoved in your spine! In case you don't know, an epidural is when a catheter is inserted via needle through the space between the vertebrae to allow for a continuous drip of anesthetic which effectively limits pain below the insertion site. In my case, the anesthetic I received was Morphine.

As we waited for the epidural placement, I decided I should try and go pee because I knew it would be much easier to do now than it would after the surgery. I got up and walked over to the bathroom. Once I started to move my gown to the side so I could do my business, I noticed that at some point the knot I tied in the back had come loose and when walking to the bathroom I gave the rest of the morning's surgery patients a view of my naked ass. I can't say I planned on giving a free show to people that morning! You've got to love those surgical gowns.

* * *

Referral For Surgery – Retroperitoneal Node Dissection Complete

I tied a much more secure knot and walked back to the curtain where I was previously and sat with my dad. Soon after, the nurse who would be inserting the epidural entered and drew the curtain and I was told to sit on the side of the bed as the nurse began to poke specific places on my spine and between my vertebrae. With my dad and a nursing student looking on, the nurse numbed the area with a local anesthetic where she decided the epidural would be placed. Once I was numb, she inserted the needle of the epidural in to the space between two vertebrae in my middle back. I don't remember the pain being too bad because my back was numb, but mostly because I was drugged for about three weeks after that point as well. I do remember, however, that I squeezed my dad's hand as I felt the needle slowly penetrate my skin and muscle and enter the synapse of my spine. From what I remember, I squeezed my dad's hand so hard that I popped one of his knuckles. I think I squeezed so hard because I anticipated immense pain knowing that something was going into my spine, not because it was actually painful. I really can't say if it was painful or not. I do not remember it being so.

The time had arrived. With an epidural in my back and an IV in my hand, I hugged my dad good-bye and walked into the surgical room. I immediately recognized the surroundings of a surgical room: the metallic equipment, the eerily sterile everything, the cold and hard surgical table. I laid myself on the table of cold metal and waited in anticipation for the nurses to cover me in the warmed blankets they keep for such occasions. Once I was comfortable (or at least as comfortable as one could get) and the medical team was ready, the anesthesiologist entered the room and said he was now going to administer the anesthesia. "Bring it on!" I thought. I knew what to expect by now and I was looking forward to seeing how long I could delay the inevitable once again. Surgeries were becoming more like a game to me rather than a lifesaving necessity. "Twenty," I began. "Nineteen. Eighteen. Seventeen. Sixthee. Fi..." I was out.

* * *

Referral For Surgery – Retroperitoneal Node Dissection Complete

A Little Mid-Surgery Surprise

I wouldn't find out until later, but this surgery didn't go exactly as planned. Dr. Sokoloff expected the surgery to be 4 hours long from first incision to last staple, but the surgery actually went on for an additional unprecedented 5 ½ hours for a total of 9 ½ hours. If you recall, I had two tumors; one in my right hip and one in my upper abdomen. Dr. Sokoloff thought that the tumor in my upper abdomen would be the most difficult of the two to remove because it was so close to my heart and major arteries, and because there are nerves in every male's abdomen that are responsible for ejaculation. If these nerves were cut, I would no longer be able to have kids naturally.

In fact, the second tumor was the reason for the lengthy procedure. None of my doctors could tell from my CT scans, PET scans, etc. that the tumor in my right hip had actually grown in and around several of the nerves sprouting out from my sciatic nerve (the large nerve that runs down both legs). My doctor was faced with a critical decision when he discovered this dilemma: 1) He could cut through the nerves thus sparing him and the rest of the surgical team an extra 5 ½ hours of surgery while virtually guaranteeing the removal of every cancer cell. However, cutting through the nerves would permanently paralyze my right leg. 2) He could take the extra 5 ½ hours and carefully dissect the tumor in an attempt to spare as many nerves as possible, thus sparing my ability to walk.

I am very grateful that Dr. Sokoloff chose the latter option. After nine hours of surgery my two tumors were gone; along with all of the lymph nodes in my back. Where would I be today if my surgeon decided he didn't want to work as hard as he did? I would be permanently confined to a wheel chair or crutches. Sure there are worse things that could have happened to me, but if I couldn't walk simply because my surgeon was lazy, I would never be able to forgive him for that. I feel so incredibly blessed to have had Dr. Sokoloff as my surgeon.

• • •

Referral For Surgery – Retroperitoneal Node Dissection Complete

Waking Up From Being Under

As I began to wake up from the anesthesia I could hear voices around me. "Is that mom? Dad? Andrea (my sister)? God?" I asked myself. I can't even begin to describe the disembodiment one feels when coming back into consciousness when previously under heavy anesthesia. You can't comprehend what is going on around you, where you are, how to respond; however, you don't even care. You simply tend to "go with the flow". A bomb could detonate right next to you and you could not care less as you mutter, "What was that? Did something just happen? Oh, a bomb. Cool." I think I got a pretty good idea of what the 60's were like.

One thing I do remember from waking up were the first words I said to my family around me. "Can I still have kids?" I asked. I so badly want(ed) to be able to have kids that those first five words reflected my concerns despite just coming out of surgery. "Yes," my mom replied as she touched my forehead. I snapped back and groaned, "No! I don't care what you say. I want to know what the doctors say!" My parents tell me the next thing I asked was, "Are there any cute nurses? I want a sponge bath." As you can probably tell, the drugs I was on made me very irritable and uninhibited.

I would come to learn much later that I was much grumpier than I realized, but I can still only think of one other time that I was rude. I remember flipping my mom off when she told me that it was getting late and she, my, dad, and my sister were going back to the hotel. I'm sure as you read this you have the same reaction as am having now as I type: "Why would he (I) be so mean, especially when nothing mean was said? What an asshole!" After talking to several nurses, I learned that such reactions are common for patients who have been under anesthesia for as long a time as I was. The best explanation given to me was, "Your mind and body have gone through a lot in a very short period of time. Your mind and body are on the defensive, and the result is often and very defensive/rude attitude; commonly one of which is

* * *

uncharacteristic for the patient." I still feel bad for how rude I was because I'm sure there were other instances that I still don't know about. My dad told me that my sister said to him, "Ok, I'll give him a few days but if he keeps acting like this I going to kick his ass!"

As I began to be more aware of my surroundings that night I got out of surgery, I was able to semi-coherently answer the questions my doctors and family had for me. That growing awareness turned out to be a godsend as I was able to find my "Magic Button;" the button to personally dispense Morphine as I deemed necessary.

So, there I was, growing in consciousness in my private hospital room with my loving family hovered around me. As I tried to carry a conversation, I stopped talking and a sudden unsettled feeling in my stomach soon was evident to those around me as my face showed a clear sign of discomfort.

"What's wrong, Brad" my dad asked.

I tried to speak, but I couldn't find the words in my brain to describe what was wrong. Finding the words felt like a chore and I was growing impatient with myself because I knew what was about to happen, yet I couldn't tell my family why I was starting to panic. Finally, I gathered all of what little energy I had and grunted, "Sick!"

Just in the knick of time, my dad quickly grabbed a nearby plastic bin and placed it on my chest as he lifted my head for me. Right on cue I began to heave, and pouring out of my mouth was the worst tasting, runny, black fluid I could ever imagine. My body continued to reject the vile substance without offering me a chance to breathe. I felt like I was going to suffocate. After what seemed to be an eternity, I finally spit out the residual fluid to try and get rid of the horrible taste left in my mouth. I had just thrown-up a dreadful mix of stomach acid, blood, and bile that had accumulated in my stomach during my nine hours of surgery.

Evidently, I didn't move to the plastic bin soon enough because a nurse who walked in during the midst of my sickness began changing my hospital gown and bedding that was drenched

• • •

in the throw-up that missed the bin. I had no idea that I was covered in the liquid and would have continued not knowing if I were the only one in the room at the time. That is how out of it I was coming to after being under for so long. You could be covered in a pile of God-knows-what and continue to not have a care in the world.

I vaguely remember the phone call, but Marisa called my room to see how I was doing. Marisa was calling from the Green Room of a concert at which our choir, The Choir of the West, was performing. At this point, my family had left for the hotel to get some sleep after a long day of waiting and doing absolutely nothing. (Can you believe there wasn't a single news stand at the hospital to keep them occupied?) I'm surprised I found the phone on the wall considering my state of mind, but I managed to do so and I found Marisa on the other end. If someone were to offer me a billion dollars to tell them what Marisa and I talked about, I wouldn't be able to do so. I only remember finding the phone. The only reason I know it was Marisa I was talking to is because she told me later that we did in fact talk that night. I suppose some advice everybody can take from my experience is to make sure you don't make any important decisions while under anesthesia and/or while connected to a bottomless bag of Morphine.

I Spent A Year In The Hospital One Week

For any night in my life I complained about not getting enough sleep, I think I made up for it while at OHSU for seven days. I guess I slept for roughly sixteen to twenty hours in both of my first two days after surgery. In the remaining five days, I would guess I slept about twelve to sixteen hours each day.

These long episodes of sleep were not over the course of long periods of time, however; far from it. Being in a hospital room with nothing to do but try and conjure up the attention span to watch TV, my mind tried to keep itself occupied. I found that was the case as every fifteen minutes or so I would wake up just in time to hear the very faint "beep" of the timer on the machine that dispensed Morphine in to my body. I learned to predict the timer so I could press the "Magic Button" and give myself the maximum dose of drugs without any interruption in-between doses. It is important to realize that this wasn't an addiction, rather a necessity because of the amount of pain I was in. I mean, seriously; you'd be doing the same thing if your entire abdomen was ripped open, internal organs removed and tossed around, and put back in place.

There were other times too when I was not able to sleep. Every day, a nurse would enter the room and cheerfully ask the same question: "So, are you ready to take a walk?" Each time I heard a nurse ask that I wanted to slap them across the room and probably would have if I could have moved. Starting on the day after my surgery I was required to walk a full circle around the wing of the hospital. This was for several reasons. They didn't want me to get bad bed sores; they didn't want my muscles to get "lazy," blah, blah, blah, blah, blah.

I'm sure it doesn't take you long to figure out why I hated the idea of walking. Let's think about this. My abdomen had been cut open and was being held together by fifty-eight staples; my stomach, large and small intestines, and kidneys are all traumatized from the surgery; and to top it all off, I am high on morphine! Each time I was supposed to "go for a walk" I had to roll over on my right side so it would be easier for me to sit up. Once I sat up, I had to grab the hands of the nurse to help me stand. Finally, once I was standing, I had to attempt to walk while drugged and return to my bed where I did the previous steps in reverse.

At first glance this probably doesn't sound like much of a challenge at all. However, what muscles are used to roll, stand, walk, sit, and lay down? That's right! Your abs! And if you'll recall, my abs were cut down the middle to get to the tumors on the lining of my back and held together by fifty-eight staples. Every time I was forced to roll over, sit up, stand, walk, and sit down, I could feel each individual staple pull against my skin. It felt as if my mid-section was tearing and soon all of my innards would spill all over the floor.

Once I began walking, I tried to complete the circle as fast as possible so the pain would be over quicker. Unfortunately, the

* * *

Referral For Surgery – Retroperitoneal Node Dissection Complete

Morphine either didn't know or didn't accept the meaning of the term "quick." I told myself to move faster, but my body would sharply reject such an order. So, with IV pole in hand being used as a walker to support myself, I slowly moved across the hospital wing six inches at a time. Moving my feet didn't hurt so much, but each time I had to shift my body weight from step to step I could once again feel the staples resist my movement and pull against one another.

When I finally completed my lap, I made my way into a chair in the corner next to my bed which felt like a blessed relief from the pain I just put myself through. There was something about resting in that chair. Yes, I was sitting up, but doing so was painless. I think that because the position of my body in the chair was different than that of when in the bed, resting in a new position offered a brief sense of relief to my body. Be that as it may, the comfort only lasted so long. After approximately ten minutes or so, I forced myself to stand up once again and lay myself once again in my bed.

Ritualistically, once I made it to that chair in the corner, another nurse would enter the room and give me a sponge bath so dead skin wouldn't pile up on my body. Honestly, I think the sponge bath was mostly for the staff's sake rather than mine. I can only imagine how bad patients would begin to smell if they weren't cleaned often.

To be perfectly honest, the seven days I was in the hospital recuperating from my surgery wasn't all that bad. I mean, I was on a twenty-four hour drug trip that felt absolutely amazing, I didn't have any work I had to do, and people were waiting on me hand and foot! There was one thing, though, that I hated and caused endless discomfort that the morphine couldn't help with. I was not allowed to eat or drink anything for the first five of the seven days I was there!

Evidently, when your internal organs go through a lot of trauma, as mine did during surgery, they shut down and take some time to get going again. So, my digestive system turned itself off

● ● ●

and if any food entered, it would just sit there and rot, causing some pretty adverse health reactions.

The hunger pains of the first two days were the worst, but as time went on (as when I didn't eat during my fourth round of chemotherapy) the pains subsided. The reason not being allowed to eat or drink was the worst part of my stay is because my mouth would get so unbelievably dry. I don't know if the dry mouth was caused by the morphine, the absence of food and liquid, or both. Whatever the cause, having a dry mouth was more of an uncomfortable nuisance than I had ever imagined. To help with the dry mouth, I was allowed one solitary ice chip each hour. A real treat.

To this day I am still trying to decide if the ice chip was a blessing or a curse. Sure, the cold ice relieved all of the discomfort I was having, but only momentarily. Once I swallowed the refreshing coolness, my mouth would begin to dry once again. Instead of having to live with a very dry mouth, I now had to live with having a very dry mouth and knowing how great it felt not to have it. The ice chip was a double edged sword. It offered temporary bliss and soon after brought even a worse sense of dry mouth, knowing I could relieve my pain, but not having the permission to do so. It was like giving a homeless man a million dollars for a week and then telling him he must go back living the life he lived before.

On the sixth day in the hospital, I was finally granted the option of eating three meals a day. I thought it was kind of funny they offered me three meals a day after having the surgery I had, plus having not been allowed to eat for the past five days. Three full meals seemed like an all-you-can-eat buffet to me! My stomach had shrunken to I don't know how small, but small enough for a few bites to make me feel plenty full. "They are just taunting me now" I'd think to myself. "Before, I wasn't given anything to eat; now they're giving me way more than I can possibly consume!" I know there must have been a method to their madness, but I definitely didn't understand it.

• • •

Referral For Surgery – Retroperitoneal Node Dissection Complete

Every day was like the last; several hours of sleep, a painful walk around the hospital wing, a sponge bath (usually by a non-English speaking nurse), and visits from my family. That was, of course, until the seventh day; the day I checked out.

Nerve Damage

I can't say I remember when Dr. Sokoloff came to visit me. I was told he came in and talked to me very early in the morning. The early hour in addition to my morphine trip didn't help me remember him visiting, I'm sure! What I do remember is talking to him, and his student whom followed him on his morning rounds, and him saying that he believed that the nerve sparing part of the surgery was a success. What did this mean? If you can recall, it meant that assuming the chemo therapy didn't permanently kill my sperm production, I should be able to ejaculate and naturally have children later on. I was very happy to hear this wonderful news.

Since I wasn't aware of the complications with the tumor in my hip, I was surprised to hear that he had to cut some nerves. Be that as it may, I was (and am) very thankful that he spent so much time to preserve the functions of my leg. I was never told that there were potential side effects from having to cut through some nerves in my hip; probably because he thought he had spared enough for there not to make a difference. Be that as it may, I did experience some "shocking" side effects.

Toward the end of my stay in the Portland hospital I began to feel what felt like electricity shoot from my knee down through my toes. The shock would always come without warning and in reaction to it, my leg would kick wildly. To describe the pain as an electric shock is the only way I can think to illustrate it. I suppose I could say it was like a knife stabbing, but the pain was not stationary; it raced down my leg, past my calf, and out my toes.

The first time it happened I was so concerned that I called for a nurse and in a panic and begged to know what was wrong with me. She had no explanation for what it could have been. She rode it off as restlessness from being confined to a bed for so long;

* * *

Referral For Surgery – Retroperitoneal Node Dissection Complete

"restless leg syndrome" she called it. I came to the conclusion that it wasn't restless leg syndrome because the shocks randomly persisted. I would later learn that the pain was coming from my nerve endings regenerating, trying to connect to where they once were.

Doctor's Notes

The patient has minimal nerve discomfort and neuropathy associated with the resection, but it was quite involved. He is doing well now. Energy has improved. The appetite seems to be getting better slowly. He has had no infection problems.

When I was finally home, and on far fewer pain killers, I noticed that the inside of my right leg was completely numb from my knee all the way to my toes (exactly where the electric shocks were occurring). The area was numb, but when I touched my calf, no matter how slightly, a great pain arose. The pain was another which I cannot begin to describe accurately. It wasn't incapacitating, rather, more annoying than anything else. However, the annoying sensation was so intense that the best way to describe it is as a pain.

As the months passed, I noticed that the shocks of sudden pain occurred far less frequently, the numbness was beginning to cover a smaller area, and finally the electric jolts subsided completely. I have read that if one's nerve endings are indeed regenerating, it can take up to ten years for them to do so completely. At the time of this writing, five years after the surgery, only a one foot vertical section of my inner right calf remains numb. I am very thankful that they are trying to regenerate, but as I tell everybody when I talk about my leg, "If I have to live with a little numbness in my leg for the rest of my life, it's a small price to pay to be cancer free.

● ● ●

Referral For Surgery – Retroperitoneal Node Dissection Complete

Going Home

There was a different sense about the nursing staff that entered my room that day. Each nurse would comment on how it was my last day and how excited I must feel to get to be going home. They were right! I was very excited to get to be going home, but it was strange to hear the excitement in their voice. I have narrowed the reasoning of their excitement down to two very opposite possibilities. Either they were trying to be supportive of my progress, or I was much ruder than I realized, and they were very happy to see me leave. I hope the former is true and not the latter.

It was only on that last day that I learned exactly how many tubes I had in my body and where they were going in and coming out! I knew about the epidural in my back that fed my Morphine. I also knew about the catheter in my penis, although I didn't know how they got it in there (they put it in when I was in surgery), nor how they planned on taking it out. I also found that I had a tube coming out of the front of my right hip. I later learned this tube drained excess fluid from my body that was created in reaction to the surgery. And, I also had an IV in my right hand where hydration was constantly dripping into my blood stream. It was time to remove all these tubes so I could go home.

"Let's start with the catheter first, ok?" the nurse asked me. I agreed but didn't really think it was going to be an enjoyable experience regardless of the order the tubes were removed. She assured me that the process wasn't going to hurt and we went on our way although I thought she was full of crap. She asked me to inhale and then exhale, and as I exhaled, she gently pulled out the catheter. I don't think there are words to describe what it feels like to have a catheter removed. All I can say is that it doesn't hurt, but it for damn sure isn't comfy! I kept exhaling until the entire catheter was finally out and I felt my eyes cross, not knowing what to think of what I was feeling. It felt like my crotch was on fire or being stung by hundreds of fire ants. The stinging was unbelievable.

* * *

Referral For Surgery – Retroperitoneal Node Dissection Complete

She then progressed on to remove the draining tube exiting my right hip. "No worries, this too won't hurt" she said soothingly. Now I thought she was really full of crap. I inhaled and exhaled once again and on my exhale, she began to slowly remove the drainage tube. This was a different sensation altogether. It was the same in the sense that it was a feeling nobody could ever be able to describe, but different because I could actually feel every inch of the tube sliding out of my gut. It felt like a snake; coiled up inside of me, searching for a way out, I could feel what felt like bumps in the tube sliding out of me. Again, there is no way to accurately describe the feelings, but it seemed like it would never end. It felt like there must have been at least ten feet of tubing inside of me although I knew there couldn't have been more than a few inches.

Both the IV in my hand and the epidural catheter in my spine were removed painlessly. Each were slid out and the tiny hole that remained was covered with a cotton swab and Band-Aid. Since I was no longer connected to my saving grace (the Morphine), I knew it wouldn't be long before I would be in a world of pain. Thankfully, the doctors sent me home with a bottle of Vicodin to hold me over on the ride home.

I waited for my mother to come to the hospital and drive me home. I think it was another hour or two until my mom finally arrived, but I didn't mind the wait. I figured if I could manage being in the hospital for seven days, I could manage to wait another couple of hours. When my mom arrived, I saw the light at the end of the tunnel. I knew I was just moments away from being freed from the building that only let me know pain and the helpless feeling of being drugged and imprisoned. I was escorted in a wheelchair to the front entrance of the hospital where a nurse and I waited for my mother to pull up the car. I was stunned by what I saw as I sat in my wheelchair; sky. Although my room did have a window, either the blinds were closed the entire time I was there, or I was too out of it to notice life outside my room. The sight of sky was all I needed at that moment to feel pain free.

• • •

Referral For Surgery – Retroperitoneal Node Dissection
Complete

I can remember the day exactly as it was. There was a brilliant canvas of blue on which a few fluffy white clouds were painted. The warm sun shone down and gently radiated warmly on my body. I sat there peacefully as I effortlessly embraced the heavenly feeling of being out of my room, out of that wing of the hospital, somewhere new. In addition to seeing sky, I also breathed in fresh air. If for only a moment, every ounce of pain I felt disappeared as my body filled with life. I gazed upon the beauty of the day and smiled.

The nurse and I watched as my mom's silver Acura pulled up and parked right in front of where we were waiting. The nurse wheeled me to my mom's car and I felt the brisk cool air that fills the Northwest in early December. At that moment, I felt more alive than I had in a very long time. My senses were overwhelmed by the sight of the sun, the bite of the cool air, the smells of winter, and the knowledge of finally being free from the hospital's sterile enclosure.

Yes, I was still in an extraordinary amount of pain, but for a brief period of time, if only for a moment, I felt like I had died and gone to Heaven. As quickly as I went into my state of bliss I plummeted back to reality when I had to climb out of the wheelchair and into my mom's waiting car. Once again I could feel my staples pulling against my skin (by now, I was no longer worried about my guts falling out and spilling onto the ground). The car was lower to the ground than the bed and chair in my room had been, so it was difficult to direct myself into the seat. Frustrated at the situation, I decided I would bite the bullet and I simply flung myself into the car. I landed forcefully onto the leather and the pain was crushing. I lifted my legs in as well and my mom shut the door behind me.

I was in so much disbelief as to the pain I just put myself through getting in the car that I couldn't even react. I flexed every muscle in my body to try and counter the feeling of torn flesh. I was able to hide my reaction to a few tears that gathered in the corner of each eye. I then inquisitively lifted my shirt to discover a trickle of blood oozing out from each side of every staple from my

* * *

sternum down to my belly button. I was too exhausted to care about a little bit of blood, so I allowed my shirt to absorb and stop the bleeding.

My mother then opened the driver's side door and I could hear her offering her thanks to the nurse who wheeled me out to her. She got into the car and we began the three hour drive home. Besides for a few speed bumps my mom took a little too quickly, the ride was pretty peaceful. That is of course once I popped three Vicodin, not having the epidural on which to rely any longer. I did have to lay the back of the seat down after a few minutes of driving because I realized I no longer had any abdominal strength to support myself while sitting up. With the seat back down and the Vicodin beginning to take effect, I passed out and didn't wake up until I was home once again.

6. *Duck Hunting – Part 1 Conclusion*

One Stubborn S.O.B.

I was so excited to be home! I was looking forward to sleeping in my own bed, not being in the confines of a sterile environment, eating. When I walked inside (albeit slowly), I plopped myself on my parent's soft, leather couch and just watched TV and took another Vicodin. It wasn't before too long that I wanted to go to bed; it was a very busy day, after all.

The next two weeks were pretty uneventful. I sat around all day every day, mostly just eating, watching TV, and sleeping. Normally, I would love to have such a break, but to be perfectly honest, I hated every minute of it. I had already had a break of over two months by this time, and I just wanted to do something new; something active.

As I've said before and as you may be able to tell by now, I'm the type of guy who refuses to accept limitations. If I'm told I can't do something or won't be able to accomplish something, I am motivated even more than before to do so. In this case, nature was telling me I couldn't do anything but stay on that damn couch. I wasn't even one week out of the hospital, two weeks out of surgery when I told my dad I wanted to go hunting that weekend.

I could tell my dad wasn't thrilled about the idea, but I insisted that we didn't let my condition get in the way of doing something we both loved. That Friday, my dad called Corky (the owner of our duck hunting club) and let him know we'd be down the next morning. Although I didn't want any special accommodations, my dad asked Corky if we could hunt out of the "Hilton" blind. This blind was the shortest walk in the whole club and would therefore be much easier for me to get to. The walk to the Hilton is only about 100 yards. Compared to the "Regency" (the longest walk in the club at roughly three quarters of a mile) it was much easier to get to. Corky agreed that the Hilton would be reserved for us.

Duck Hunting – Part 1 Conclusion

The next morning, we woke up at 4:00am and drove an hour and fifteen minutes south to the Lincoln Creek Duck Club in Rochester, Washington, a rural area just outside of Chehalis, WA. When we reached the club, I eased out of my dad's Ford F-150 truck, careful not to hurt myself since the truck is somewhat high off the ground. My dad had to carry my chest waders and jacket in for me because I wasn't supposed to lift anything heavy. Carrying my gear in addition to his, it was hard not to laugh as he could barely see above it all.

We entered the local Grange Hall where all members met to be assigned a blind for that day's hunt. Taking tiny steps I could feel everybody's eyes on me. All of the members knew what I had been going through and I think they were surprised beyond belief that I was actually going to hunt when at that time one week earlier I was in a hospital recovering from my surgery. I had been hunting with many of these men since I was 13 years old, so they had seen be grow up over the years. It's understandable they were concerned for my well-being. I pretended not to notice all the attention and said hello to everybody there as if everything was normal.

Normally, it was at that time when I would pull on my waders. Being the overly proud person I am, I tried to do so on my own but as I tried, I felt my staples begin to pull and I quickly grabbed my belly. I had no choice but to ask for my dad's help. As he helped me slide on my right boot and then my left, I refused to feel embarrassed that I couldn't even dress myself. Actually, I felt proud. Not that I couldn't dress myself of course, but proud that I wasn't letting my cancer/surgery get in the way of living. I thought to myself, "Yeah, that's right! I can't dress myself. But I'm alive and I'm here. I'm doing what I love to do despite just coming out of surgery!" I even think I cracked a small smile as my dad pulled up the last bit of neoprene. It is strange when you get these brief moments of empowerment and pride. I never thought one would come when I helplessly couldn't dress myself in a room full of rugged hunters!

● ● ●

Duck Hunting – Part 1 Conclusion

Once we left the Grange and parked to where we could begin walking to the Hilton, my dad helped me put on my camouflaged jacket weighed down by two pockets filled with shotgun shells. I wanted to carry a bag of decoys on my back as I normally would have, but even I knew that wasn't possible. Luckily, Corky assigned another man to hunt with us that day, so he carried them instead. Although I wasn't supposed to carry anything, I refused to let anybody carry my gun for me. Once again, I wanted to keep some bit of independence, no matter how little it was. We waded through standing water to the blind, set out the decoys, and got settled in the blind as we waited for the legal shooting time to come.

I felt perfectly fine for the first hour or so besides a little tenderness along my staples. The hunting was slow as we didn't have many ducks flying in the early part of the morning just before sunrise. As the minutes passed I began to feel aches growing up and down my back. I didn't want to say anything because I knew my dad would be concerned and say we should probably go home. Instead, I nonchalantly rested my elbows on my knees easing some weight of my back. I toughed it out for another thirty minutes or so until I broke down and told my dad how bad my back was feeling. I insisted that we continue hunting and I would just lie down on the bench for a while to alleviate all of the weight. He reluctantly agreed and I turned to lie down.

Here's a challenge for you. Ready? I want you to try and lie down and not flex your abs on the way down. Go ahead. Try it. Can you do it? My guess is you can't. Now, imagine doing that with your abs split open and fifty-eight staples pulling every which way. As I leaned back to lie down I instinctively tried to flex my abs to control the speed at which I leaned back, and as my muscles failed I went falling backwards. My back landed with a thud and I was overwhelmed with all sorts of pain.

"Ooohhh! Are you okay, Brad?" my dad asked. At this point in the book you probably have a good idea of what my answer was. I lied to him as tears gathered in my eyes and said with a slight laugh, "Oh, yeah. No problem." I continued to lie

●　●　●

there for a while and concentrated on not letting the pain intensify. After only a few minutes I had to sit up again. I just couldn't get rid of the pain growing by the minute.

I slowly rolled off of the bench and on to my knees where I then was able to sit myself on the bench with relatively little pain. After only another few minutes the pains in my back returned. Swallowing my pride, I finally turned to my dad and said, "Dad, I'm sorry but I think I need to go home." He was more than happy to go since he knew I was in pain, and I don't think he wanted me there in the first place. We apologized to our hunting partner for having to leave early, but he wouldn't accept an apology. He understood that I was in pain and helped us pack up our things. We had only been in the field for a little over two hours and I had to go home. When we got to the truck, my dad helped me take off my waders and I climbed in and immediately reclined the seat.

I look back to that day and I can't help but smile. I now realize that I had begun to live my life then how I do now. I refuse to wait until tomorrow to live. If I want to do something, I will find a way to do it. Why? Because I want to. It is as simple as that. That is the only reason I need. You will read much more about this in the second section of this book, but I learned that I can't take any day for granted. I am determined to live for today because tomorrow is never guaranteed. We are only promised the moment in which we live, and once any moment reaches us, it has already passed.

A Call From Dr. Sokoloff

Laying on the couch, as was my go-to position, the phone next to me rang. I answered the phone and on the other end of the line was Dr. Nichols. When he said hello my heart sank. Immediately, possible reasons for his call flew wildly through my head as I half listened to what he was saying. I gathered myself together and listened intently. "We have received the pathology report from the lymph nodes we removed in your surgery, and I am happy to tell you it looks like no living cancer cells remained.

Duck Hunting – Part 1 Conclusion

At this point nothing further is required from you. I will send a copy of the report to Dr. Senecal so he has it on file."

It sounded like good news, but I wasn't exactly sure what I was being told. "Does that mean I am cancer free?" I asked. He told me that not only was I cancer free, but I can now refer to myself as "in remission". ("Remission" is when no identifiable cancer indicating signs or symptoms exist. "Cured" is a term usually used once five years have passed from entering remission, without being re-diagnosed with cancer.) Not knowing how to react, I thanked him for the news and said goodbye.

How was I supposed to react? I was confused and questions raced through my head: "I fought this disease every day for four and a half months and all of a sudden it has just, disappeared? What do I do now? Sure, I need to have a CAT scan every three months and meet with Dr. Senecal once a month, but I'm sure there's got to be something else I need to do. Right?" What had been an exasperating battle every waking moment since I was diagnosed was now all of a sudden supposed to be an afterthought. I couldn't wrap my head around that. "How do I just flip a switch and pick up from where I left off?" I decided I would just lie back down, continue watching T.V., and continue to heal.

Removing Fifty-Eight Staples

Again, those two weeks after leaving the hospital weren't very eventful. I spent most of my time laying horizontal on the couch, trying to not rip open my belly with any sudden movements. But, at the end of those two weeks, it was finally time to get those pesky staples out of me!

My dad drove me to the office and in no time at all I was in a private room where a nurse explained how she was going to "gently ease each staple out." She told me that it doesn't really hurt, that most people say it's like a tiny tug on each staple. I thought she was full of shit. "Yeah, they're just metal tacks in my belly," I joked to myself, "why would that hurt?" Much to my surprise, and delight, she was right. There was barely any pain to speak of.

Granted I am thoroughly convinced that once you face great amounts of pain, later painful events are dulled by your past experience. The only "pain" was the slight tug she had described. The nurse slid what looked like a letter opener between my skin and the staple and gently lifted the staple out of my abdomen and into a waiting pan.

Previous worries of my skin opening up and my guts falling out all over the place flew to the forefront of my mind. As I laid on the table, I watched intently as I counted each removed staple. One... two... three... I also wanted to make sure to watch for not if, but when my insides began to spill out so I could catch them and hold them in place until help could come. Twenty-eight... twenty-nine... thirty... I was relieved after each staple came out with no pain and with no spilling organs. Forty-five... forty-six... forty-seven... I did notice tiny trickles of blood oozing out of almost every place where a stapled had been. Forty-eight... forty-nine... fifty... I didn't care about that so much, but as the nurse was reaching the last of my staples, I saw my skin begin to tear along the scar of the incision. I started to panic a little bit, but the nurse reassured me that the tearing was common and she cleaned off the area and placed two butterfly bandages across the break. Fifty-six... fifty-seven... fifty-eight... In just a matter of minutes, all the staples were removed. To insure the skin wouldn't open anywhere else, she placed Steri-Strips™ covered in an adhesive along the scar. After a few seconds of drying time, I pulled my shirt on, said thank you, and met my dad out in the lobby. It was as simple as that!

It never ceases to amaze me how whenever I was even the slightest bit apprehensive about a procedure I had to go through, my expectations were always worse than the actual experience. That is one of the main motivating reasons for me writing this book. The scariest part about having cancer is not knowing. Not knowing what to expect; not knowing if what you are feeling is normal; not knowing what everything you are being told means.

Hopefully by reading this, you as a fighter, family member of a fighter, or friend of a fighter can gain some knowledge of what you, your family member, or your friend may experience.

Surgery Number 4: Port Removal

After a week of being "stapleless" I went for my first appointment with Dr. Senecal after having had surgery. It was the same protocol as every other appointment. I waited for my name to be called in the waiting room, I was weighed, and I waited a little longer in the examination room for Dr. Senecal to arrive. The examination was also the same: I breathed in and breathed out deeply while he listened to my heart and lungs, breathed in and out deeply while he poked my belly and tapped along my back, dropped my pants so he could check for recurrent cancer in my remaining left testicle.

As I was buttoning my pants Dr. Senecal reassured me that everything checked out great. That was definitely very welcomed news. Although I was confident nothing bad was going to turn up, I was relieved to hear that I was healthy once again.

"So what's next?" I asked.

"Well, now we need to schedule a CAT scan for one month from now. Actually, we need to schedule a CAT scan for one month from now, another one for three months from then, and another for three months from then." I was surprised to find I needed all of those CTs.

I asked why it was I needed to have so many CAT scans and I was further shocked when he replied that I would need to have a CAT scan every three months for the next two years. I learned that to have so many scans after entering remission is standard practice. "We just want to be careful" Dr. Senecal explained. I had no problem being careful. Actually, I was happy to hear that he wanted to be so careful. "Better safe than sorry," I thought. Besides, it was my being careful which led to finding my cancer in the first place!

In addition to having a CAT scan every three months, I was to have an appointment with Dr. Senecal once every month for a check-up. A week before every appointment I was instructed to come in to the office and get my blood drawn as I had done so many times before. I was to have my CBC (Complete Blood Count) and my AFP (alpha-fetoprotein) counted. Just like my CAT scans, my monthly doctor appointments and blood draws were to occur for the next two whole years.

By now, for quite some time, I had gotten used to needles and had no problem getting poked month after month. Be that as it may, I was happy of the fact that I still had my port in my chest. Whenever I went to get my blood drawn, the nurse would simply access my port and take my blood from there rather than poking my arm. This made it so I continued to not feel the needle.

That luxury could only last so long, however. I scheduled to get my port removed on Thursday August 18th. It had been ten months since my last dose of chemo, and I decided I'd prefer to have the port removed before school began again. The reason I had kept the port in for so long was because my doctors told me it was better to keep it in just in-case additional chemo was needed if the cancer returned during my first year in remission. I was close to the one year mark and the port had served its purpose. It was time to get it out.

I made arrangements for me to be put under while I had the port removed. Normally, just a local anesthetic is used when removing a port. A few doctors told me that I simply wouldn't be allowed to be put under for such a simple and painless operation, but I insisted that I be unconscious for the surgery. Why was I so adamant about being put under for the surgery? Well, while reading during those long episodes of receive my chemo drugs, I read a story where a patient's port had been in his chest for so long that it had actually attached itself to his pectoral muscle and the doctors had to "tear" the port apart from the muscle. I don't know if that story is true, but I reasoned that although it is unlikely that the same thing would happen to me, I had been through enough pain during my treatment and I didn't want anymore. There was no way in Hell anybody was going to tell me I had to be awake for the surgery!

Duck Hunting – Part 1 Conclusion

As expected, the port removal surgery went without a hitch. There were no problems, it only took twenty minutes, and the port had not attached itself to my muscle. From that day forward, when I went to get blood tests, the nurses accessed my vein in my right arm since my port was gone. I remember the first time I went to get a blood test after my port was removed. I took a deep breath in anticipation for the sting I was certain to feel. But, much to my surprise, I didn't even know the needle was in my arm until I looked down and saw it there! The number of times my arm had been accessed (before I had my port) destroyed many of the nerves in the crutch of my right arm. In other words, the nerves in my arm were severed enough that I no longer feel when a needle is inserted in my arm. I knew I'd be able to deal with the needles if I had to, but I love the fact that I can't feel anything when the times come that I do need to be poked.

Scar Tissue

It was during one of those standard monthly check-ups, relatively soon after my "curing" surgery, that Dr. Senecal noticed an anomaly on my CT scan. Sitting in the examination room, he explained what he was seeing on the films. Viewing image by image I was shown an elongated piece of white (hard tissue) similar to the pictures I have come to hate. I saw where it began and where it ended; and I also saw how it did not appear on the other side of my body.

I couldn't imagine it was more cancer. "How could cancer possibly come back after going through all that chemo?" I asked myself. "It can't be cancer! I was told that the surgery was a complete success and no living cancer cells were found in my post-surgical pathology report!" In an instant I realized that I was doing exactly what I told myself I would not do while I went through my treatments. I was worrying before there was anything to worry about. I then calmed down, refocused on Dr. Senecal, and listened to what he had to say.

"Often times after surgery your body works so hard to heal itself that it does too good a job and scar tissue builds" he explained. "This is what we see here" he said pointing to the CT films. Thrilled to hear the white blip on the CT was not in fact cancer I said, "Oh, good! Nothing to worry about."

Although it is true that the scar tissue itself was harmless, the effects of it were another story. Dr. Senecal continued, "You see, this scar tissue is beginning to press against your right ureter coming from your kidney. Currently it is not a problem, but if it progresses further you may need another surgery to remove the scar tissue to prevent other potentially serious health complications."

Simply put, the ureter is a tube that carries urine from each kidney to the bladder. Since we have two kidneys we also have two ureters. The types of problems that could occur are not important for this book, and I am sure that if you happen to find yourself in a similar situation your doctor will explain everything clearly. If not, be sure to ask.

So, the good news was that I did not have a recurrence of cancer and that the scar tissue was not yet an issue. The bad news was that it was something we would need to keep a close eye on and be prepared to take action if it grew to a point of affecting my ureter. In the grand scheme of things, it wasn't bad news at all, just something to monitor.

I continued to have my check-ups every month and CAT scans every three months as I was instructed. I had no complications with doing so until I was presented with a wonderful opportunity; an internship position at the Lance Armstrong Foundation (LAF) in Austin, Texas. After having submitted an application and being interviewed, I was offered the internship and accepted it immediately. The only problem with going to Texas was that I needed a CAT scan while I was there. I also needed to find a doctor for my monthly check-up and to read the CT films.

The Lance Armstrong Foundation (LAF)

For the summer of 2005 I moved to Austin, Texas and worked as an intern with the Lance Armstrong Foundation (LAF). I was excited to work with what I assumed would be a wonderful group of people, working selflessly for a common cause, and helping the greater cancer community. All my assumptions proved to be true. I couldn't have asked to work with more caring or more committed people.

I interned in the Development Department and fellow interns worked alongside leadership in various other business units. There was typically one intern per department. Arriving at the office on the first day, the other interns and I were welcomed with a warm reception and a few presentations and words from "Team LAF" (the LAF employees). We were then shone to our work stations and given projects on which to work right away.

Working in the Development Department, my overall mission was to aid in creating a successful annual fundraising return. This goal was broken down into three specific areas of action: 1) Event Planning, 2) Fundraising, and 3) Constituent and Donor Relations. Although that was the scope of my internship position, I was in Austin solely for the purpose of helping the foundation so I offered myself as a resource that could be utilized across all departments. The internship itself offered plenty opportunity to learn, but offering to work an undefined number of hours allowed me to gain an even richer experience.

My typical day involved speaking with grassroots fundraisers across the country (and sometimes across the world); answering any questions they had, help brainstorm fundraising ideas, and deciding what collateral I could offer to help promote their events and educate others about cancer. Some days I would receive only a hand full of calls, but most days my phone would ring again as soon as I hung up the phone after speaking with another patron.

When I wasn't receiving calls I was reaching out to major donors and fundraisers from the previous two years. More often than not, these people were not in need of any assistance since they were veterans of the fundraising/donating game. For those who did have questions, I was more than happy to answer them. Whether they required assistance or not, it was an opportunity to thank them for their previous support and encourage them to continue their great work.

Speaking with these advocates was a genuinely rewarding experience. So often would they take the time to thank me for the work I was doing and describe how they first became involved with the LAF. Sure, many of the stories I listened to were sad, but a common theme I heard was regardless of the fate of their own story, they knew they could make a difference by taking action in one way or another. They knew that cancer had changed them for the better and nothing was going to prevent them from helping others affected by this horrible disease.

Finally I was in a place where people understood as I did. I often say that cancer has been the best thing that has ever happened to me. Until working at the LAF I never felt like anybody could relate to the way I felt, or they resented what I said because they had a loss due to cancer. The people with whom I spoke and those working at the foundation understood that cancer itself is not in itself a good thing. Far from it. They all knew that it is what we are able to gain from the cancer experience that is priceless; if we choose to look at it that way.

If I wasn't on the phone, I was likely working feverously to register participants for the Peloton Project. The Peloton Project (which has since grown into the much larger Livestrong Ride Series) was the annual cornerstone fundraising initiative of the Lance Armstrong Foundation. Participants would register to fundraise for the foundation and participate in the end of the year fundraising celebration, the Ride for the Roses in Austin, Texas where participants rode between 10 and 100 miles through the city on their bikes.

I would process registrants' paperwork, enter their information in the database, and assemble and mail their registration packet. Each packet included a registration card as well as various pieces of collateral and fundraising information. It may not sound like an exciting job, but the beginning of summer was when registration was at its height. I would often process a few hundred registrants a day and the real reward was looking at all of the mailings I prepared, knowing that my work would effectively help raise tens if not hundreds of thousands of dollars for the foundation.

When there was some down time, I volunteered to update the foundation's new database system. Right when my internship began, the LAF switched to a new database system and needed to input all of the donors' information into this new system. In addition to moving all of the donor information from the old system, we received hundreds of additional contacts daily from various community events and new registrants for the Peloton Project. I saw this as an opportunity to really make a sizable contribution to the foundation itself when I had extra time to spare. As I painstakingly entered the seemingly endless names, numbers, addresses, etc., I became quite proficient with the program. Before I knew it, I was the go-to person when anybody had a question about how to most effectively and efficiently use the new software.

Perhaps the most exciting times of my internship were the Tour de Lance parties which the LAF threw in restaurants and bars throughout downtown Austin. My internship took place while Lance Armstrong was pursuing his unprecedented seventh Tour de France win. We would watch stages of the Tour every day in the office, but on the weekend of the 23rd and 24th of July, 2005 the LAF threw parties in downtown Austin so fans could celebrate Lance's win as a community.

We sold LAF merchandise to the fans, provided educational material, and recruited even more fundraisers to help support the LAF cause. It was much less an opportunity to make money for the Foundation than it was an opportunity to bring the community together to celebrate one of their own. The atmosphere was electric with proud sports fans, cancer survivors, and the general public in attendance as well as local news crews and radio stations.

However, the reason these two days were so exciting for me was more than the celebratory feel in the air. On the Friday before the parties were to take place I was asked by the LAF's

Media Relations manager if I would mind being interviewed by one of the local news channels. "They would like to talk about the Tour de Lance parties and I thought it would be great to have the LAF represented by a cancer survivor such as yourself" she said. I agreed to do the interview (really... was I going to pass up this opportunity?) and she replied, "Great! You will be interviewed tomorrow at 6am. Let's discuss what to expect."

She spent an hour with me, giving me a crash course in how to speak with the media. We discussed key speaking points as well as the appropriate way to answer a question so it is easier for the news team to edit the interview for broadcast. Armed with this new bit of knowledge we agreed to meet at five o'clock the next morning to begin setting up the first restaurant for the party and to prepare for the interview.

I arrived the next morning with coffee in hand (I don't think I can live without my morning latte) excited for the parties and interview to come. I was not anxious at all for the interview. In my mind I had nothing to be nervous about. However, ten minutes before the interview was to be shot, the reporter told me that the interview would be live. My heart immediately began to race. "What if I mess up? What if I say something wrong, or sound nervous because now I am nervous? I want to represent the LAF well and professionally. What if I don't do a good job?"

"And we're live in five, four, three..." the camera man counted. When the camera went on and I saw the live picture on the screen in front of me, most of my nerves (realize I say most of my nerves, not all) went away and I carried on an interview that lasted approximately two minutes. When the live feed went back to the anchors in the studio I let out a big exhale and the reporter, the LAF's Media Relations manager, and the other interns who were there all said I did a really good job. I was relieved to hear it went well. I found later that day that my interview must have been even better than I thought because I was asked to do three more television interviews for different networks, as well as a radio interview. I like to think that by the end of that Saturday my

* * *

interviewing skills were beginning to be fairly polished; at least as polished as I could get with one day's experience.

I should say one last thing about working with the LAF. Not only are the employees and volunteers of the foundation an incredible group of people, but they know how to have fun while they work and maintain strong workplace morale and unity not often seen in an office environment. In my experience with the LAF there was a lot of personal freedom in that there was little if any noticeable micromanaging. Also, the team atmosphere was lived rather than preached. This was evident by hosting several group lunches and gatherings after work. In general, the environment was one of hospitability, warmth, and a passion to assist the cancer community. I cannot say enough good things about the LAF and the people who work there.

Dr. "X"

To protect the identity of a doctor I mention at this point, I will refer to him as "Dr. X".

Doctor's Notes

(From Dr. Frank Senecal to "Dr. X")

Dear Doctor X:

This is a brief note to introduce you to Mr. Brad Lubken. Mr. Lubken is a patient under my care who was diagnosed with testicular cancer. He was diagnosed in the summer of 2004. He was a student at Pacific Lutheran University in Tacoma, Washington. He presented with a mass in the right testicle almost 4cms in diameter. He was found at radical orchiectomy to have a mixed germ cell tumor which included both mature teratoma and embryonal cell characteristics. His alpha-fetoprotein was over 2000. CT scans demonstrated retroperitoneal adenopathy, staging him at a 2C.

The patient was treated with systemic chemotherapy and experienced a good response to the V-16, Bleomycin, and Cisplatinum. The alpha-fetoprotein progressively regressed and we were able to document regression of adenopathy. At the end of four cycles he continued to have identifiable residual mass however in the retroperitoneum.

I referred him to Craig Nichols because of persistent elevation of the alpha-fetoprotein for consideration of rather involved surgical resection. Doctor Nichols in turn referred him to Doctor Mitchell Sokoloff at Oregon Health Sciences. Doctor Sokoloff performed a retroperitoneal node dissection removing both a right pelvic mass and right periaortic mass. This resection demonstrated residual mature teratoma in the product material. There was no viable carcinoma identified.

Since that time the patient has remained in remission. He has no evidence of recurrent disease. He is due for CT scans again for monitoring in July. Alpha-fetoprotein and beta HCGs have been normal.

I appreciate your consideration of Mr. Lubken. He will be working for the Lance Armstrong Foundation while he is in Austin and I know that you will enjoy your relationship with him.

Thank for your help.

Sincerely,

Frank M. Senecal, M.D./kp

Duck Hunting – Part 1 Conclusion

I asked Dr. Senecal if he knew of any good urologists in Austin and he later referred me to Dr. X whom had an office in North Austin. I had researched Dr. X and found he was highly respected and had built a great reputation in the area. I found where his office was located and Dr. Senecal arranged my check-up to be with him and for my CAT scan to be performed at the nearby Seton Northwest Hospital.

After finding my way to Dr. X's office I sat in the waiting room anxious to meet such a highly recommended doctor. The appointment process in this office was pretty much the same as at Dr. Senecal's; wait, be taken to a private room where vitals are taken, wait, wait some more, and finally meet the doctor for the check-up.

Having waited for only a few minutes for the doctor, the door opened and in walked Dr. X. I found myself looking at a fifty-something, average height man whose obesity radiated a staggering intimidation. He wore a pair of thin rimmed glasses, his complexion wasn't pale but light in color, and his roughly kept mustache dominated his profile. Despite his several memorable physical traits, the thing that I noticed the most, and continues to be his most memorable feature, was that he never even remotely cracked the slightest bit of a smile.

I was immediately uncomfortable in that room. I had always expected to see Dr. Senecal enter the room whose mannerisms never failed to bring calm to any anxiety one may have. It was at that moment that I realized just how fortunate I was to have Dr. Senecal as my Oncologist. Dr. Senecal was very professional, all the while paying careful attention to compassion; on the other hand, Dr. X was strictly all business.

The check-up was very quick in comparison to any other appointment I had had. He examined me and asked a few questions. I told him that I was concerned about my lungs because it was noticeably more difficult to breathe than before having chemotherapy. He told me to talk to the nurse in the infusion room to schedule a spirometer test (the same kind of test I had when I had my first round of chemo as in-patient) in addition to

* * *

my CAT scan and he left to see his next patient. I was shocked by the lack of attention I received during the appointment, but nothing could have prepared me for what I would witness next.

I went to the infusion room to schedule my spirometer test and CT, and after a few minutes I saw a lady who was receiving some chemo stand up and began talking to Dr. X, who walked in for some paperwork for another patient. The lady was clearly frightened. You could hear her concerns in her voice and see them on her face. She was asking him questions about a new cocktail of drugs he put her on. Dr. X was obviously annoyed with her and only offered quick, short answers so he could get to where he needed to go (my guess is that he wanted to be anywhere but there).

Continuing with her questions her voice got a bit louder and her tone rose with growing concern and emotion. Unexpectedly, Dr. X burst out yelling, "Don't you get it? You almost died last week! Everything we're doing for you, your body rejects it! Nothing is working!" The lady burst into tears in front of everybody in the infusion room. A friend of hers began walking her back to her chair as the lady repeatedly cried, "I don't want to die, I don't want to die…" A more collected Dr. X followed and stated, "Listen, we just want to be careful because we don't want you to have a reaction like last week's. We don't want you to go into another coma; no matter how short of one it may be."

Evidently, the lady had been having a tough time with her treatment. The chemo she was taking resulted in potentially deadly rejections from her body and they had been trying different amounts of different drugs to try and treat her cancer without killing her first.

I was appalled by quite a few things Dr. X said and did just then. First of all, a doctor should never yell or make a scene in an office. Emotions are already running rampant in an infusion room. Some people are contemplating what life and death mean to them, others may be trying to make plans for their family in case they die. Secondly, the things Dr. X said were strictly confidential and therefore should only be disclosed to others with the consent of the patient. Sure, the lady approached him in front of others, but he should have either spoken in a voice where only the two of them could hear or taken her to another room. There was no excuse for his actions.

To compare Dr. X to Dr. Senecal again, I can't picture Dr. Senecal ever making a patient cry (unless it was the result of some unfortunate news he had to deliver). The words that flew out of Dr. X's mouth convinced the lady that she was going to die. I've always thought (and continue to do so) that oncology is a profession only for those who have an utmost love for people. How else could oncologists deal with the great accomplishments and devastating defeats to which they hold witness every day?

It took all of my energy not to approach her and say, "You should never feel obligated to be with the doctor you are seeing. You are not stuck. You have every right in the world to find a doctor you trust and respect. This is your fight… use the weapons you want to use." I decided it wasn't my place to say anything. Be that as it may, I am not happy that I decided not to say anything. With some reflection, I think that as a fellow fighter/survivor, it was my place to say something. I understood what she deserved as a person fighting cancer.

I left the office happy to know I only had to see Dr. X one more time (to review my CT films) and I would never again have to be around him. I had my check-up and the information about where and when my CAT scan and spirometer test would be. I was happy to get out of that office.

The CAT scan was like every other CAT scan I've had; although I thought it was strange that the contrast that I had to drink came in glass bottles. I felt as if I was magically whisked back fifty years when all liquids came in glass. I guess Texans really do do things differently. Anyhow, I drank the chalky Barium filled substance, had my CT, took the spirometry test, and returned to the home I was renting for the summer.

When I had to go back to Dr. X's office for the films to be read, I was hoping it would be a very quick appointment so I didn't have to witness any more uncouth doctoring. Thankfully, the wait was short and (as expected) Dr. X wasn't exactly all that social. He noticed the growing scar tissue impinging on my right ureter, and I reassured him that I already knew about it, but the films needed to be sent to Dr. Senecal in Tacoma to check if it had grown any since my previous scan. Needless to say, I was happy to hear that no cancer was found in the latest set of films, but that was what I expected. When I realized I wasn't scared about the scan finding cancer, I recognized that I may be beginning to take my health for granted as I had (as we all do) before I was diagnosed; that I may have been becoming complacent in being cancer free.

The thought of not worrying about falling out of remission was, at times, scarier than when I was told I had cancer. I don't want the fear of losing my health to be lost because I'm certain that could lead to a slippery slope where I will eventually take my health for granted once again. I consider my fear a blessing not only for me, but to those with whom I am able to share that fear. If sharing my story encourages others to pay attention to their own health, you better believe I consider my fear a good thing.

Before the appointment wrapped up, Dr. X read the results of my diffusion test. It turned out that my lungs were a little below average when they diffuse oxygen into my blood stream. Be that as it may, the results weren't severe enough to suggest that the failing diffusion was the entire reason for my breathing problems. Dr. X determined that the Bleomycin I took as part of my chemo cocktail formed scar tissue on the small air sacs in my lungs called alveoli, thus constricting the amount of air my lungs could hold. When I told Dr. Senecal what Dr. X suggested, he told me that when this happens it can be permanent; that is, if the person chooses. Evidently, continuous exercise can help break-up a lot of the scar tissue and bring your lungs back to relative normality.

How I Am Today

So, how am I today? I am happy to report that I continue to remain cancer free and I am living life to the fullest. I was officially cured on October 15th, 2009 (five years after my last dose

● ● ●

of chemo). My lungs are in much better condition today, but singing still tends to be a bit difficult. However, I think that is likely because I am not active in solo or choral performances. I've made it a goal to bring my lungs back to the condition they once were by exercising regularly. It has been very hard and painful work, but I believe I am just about back to normal.

The scar tissue which had been growing against the ureter of my right kidney has not advanced any more. However, at a recent physical exam, high levels of protein were discovered in my urine which subsequently led to finding that the scar tissue has completely killed-off the kidney. It is now practically a big sack of water sitting in my side. Thankfully, my doctors tell me I can live a normal life with my other healthy kidney. But, if I develop a fever and pain in my side, it is likely that the hydronephrotic kidney has become infected and will need to be removed immediately. I'm keeping my fingers crossed that I can avoid that surgery.

Conclusion

I have said it before and I will say it again: Cancer is the best thing to have ever happened to me. I never wished for it and would never wish it upon anybody else, but the life threatening disease was a catalyst for me to learn more about myself I could have ever dreamed, and it forced me to appreciate life to an extent I could not otherwise have understood. These two lessons learned made the entire ordeal worth it. All the dropped tears, expelled vomit, bodily scars, and emotional swings were simply the price I paid for the privilege of becoming a better person. I paid that tuition, and feel like I have aced the class.

If you have cancer, are a friend or family member of somebody facing cancer, or are reading this book because you are curious about what the cancer experience is like, I hope my story has been helpful. The most important things I hope you will take away are:

Survivors are not people to be pitied. Survivors are people; treat them as such. One of the quickest ways to make them feel defeated is to give them "special" treatment. Trust me, they are getting plenty special treatment in the chemo ward.

The best thing you can do for a survivor is simply be there for them. Invite them to join you on errands, go to parties, go drinking. As was the case with me, I just wanted to feel like everything was normal. What may seem like an insignificant gesture to you may very well mean the world to somebody facing the fight of and for their life.

Make life happen. I sincerely hope you don't have to go through cancer or any other life threatening ordeal to learn to appreciate life. I hope my words will encourage you to see the good in things even when the good is not obvious. I hope my words will encourage you to take control of your life and make good things happen rather than wait for good things to happen to you. And, I hope my words will encourage you maintain a positive attitude when times get tough, because that positivity just may be your deciding factor.

I thank you for taking the time to read what I faced before, during, and after my cancer experience. It is a very moving story for me, and for you as well, I hope. While writing this book, I focused on being as accurate as possible while also being entertaining. If you laughed, gasped, and/or reflected throughout this first half of the book, my mission has been completed.

I strongly encourage you to continue reading through to the end of the book. Whereas Part 1 focused on my experience before, during, and after cancer; Part 2 concentrates on what I have learned about life while battling cancer. In many ways Part 2 is more important than Part 1. The choice is yours, but I am sure you will be happy you read on. Besides, it's much shorter than Part 1. Go on… you know you want to!

Part 2

1. *Intro*

As we march through the never-ending adventure of life, it is clear that as rational beings we mature. Maturity involves change but it does not mean we change who we are; rather we alter how it is we express who we have found we are to be. Like anybody else, I went through several changes. In retrospect I can identify two pivotal changes in my life. The first was when I made the leap from being a strongly introverted child to a fairly extroverted young adult. The second was when I went from being a self-doubting, glass is half-empty individual to an excessively optimistic life loving fanatic.

As a child I was very shy. I cannot find the words to adequately describe how shy I was. I would speak quietly and mumble, walk hunched over with my head always looking down, and never approach somebody I didn't know. As you can imagine, I was the one usually picked last at recess and would often isolate myself from recess play, finding a corner where I would sit alone and listen to music until the whistle blew to go back to class. My shyness led to a self-inflicted painful childhood. (It is important to emphasize that the pain was strictly self-inflicted. I didn't realize it at the time, but I was choosing to be shy and antisocial. I had the best parents anybody could ask for, so my home life was wonderful. It was my interaction with my peers that was the problem.) However, two specific events in the eighth and ninth grade were the defining moments of when I turned extrovert.

In eighth grade I ran for Curtis Junior High School ASB Senator in University Place, WA. As a shy kid, I prepared a short speech and presented it in front of the entire junior high school. I was nowhere near brave enough to do something funny and non-traditional (which, of course, is how you get elected in that kind of thing). Once the assembly was over, and my heart rate finally dropped below 300 beats per minute, the results of the election came in. And surprise surprise, I wasn't elected. The next year I decided to run again but I convinced myself to work up the

• • •

courage to do something drastically out of character for that speech. I knew that if I wanted to win the election I would have to shock the audience. I also knew that I hated living the shy life I had always lived. It was time for a change.

I memorized the popular sketch from Saturday Night Live where comedian Chris Farley played motivational speaker Matt Foley who lived "in a van down by the river." I dressed in a fat suit and looked just like the character on SNL. I even made a table out of balsa wood on which I threw myself upon, just like Chris Farley. The words of the sketch were almost exactly like the original, only altered to make sense for the election. As I picked myself up from the shattered balsa wood table at the end of my speech, the auditorium erupted in deafening applause. This time the results were different; I was elected. Seeing the reaction to my speech I realized that I could feel comfortable in front of groups and so I began to stray from shyness.

I tell you this story because I want to show what I mean by changes in life. Pivotal changes can be sudden like my change from introvert to extrovert or gradual as well. This second half of my book is meant to describe how I have changed from pessimist to optimist; the second pivotal change I mentioned. Even more so, I want to explain what I have learned via my bout with cancer and how it has helped me learn to appreciate life much more than I ever knew possible. It is my hope that by reading the following chapters you will choose to incorporate what I have learned into your own life as much as possible and benefit as I have.

Before reading on, you should know that because I am talking about life lessons I have learned from my cancer experience, the writing can come off as a bit philosophical at times. Do not let that stop you. I promise that the lessons I've learned will improve your life dramatically if you allow them to.

2.   *Optimism, Pessimism, Realism*

Prior to being diagnosed on July 30th, 2004, I rarely if ever paid careful attention to the attitude of those around me, let alone my own. I had little interest in noticing the reactions of others, probably because I didn't have the perspective I do now. I was young in age and in experience, and found no benefit of focusing on such things. Frankly, I was more interested in my own hobbies and sports; the typical things a high school/new college student was interested in. It never crossed my mind to carefully consider how my reactions to situations affect me or how other's reactions affect those around them as well.

To be honest, before I was diagnosed with cancer I was the person I have come to despise. I was a loyal member of the "Pessimism Party". It was common for me to complain about any given situation, to blame my problems on others, and to never see the good or the potential good in a bad situation. Looking back at myself, I would have never wanted to be around me. My approach to life was extremely self-defeating which brought dissatisfaction along with it; which brings me to the point of this chapter.

People now say they respect my outlook on life, but that I am "over the top" and unrealistic. To justify their moments of negativity they say, "I'm not being pessimistic, just realistic!" I've become gripped by this statement and I have questioned myself over and over; what is the difference between optimism, pessimism, and realism? We all need to have a clear understanding of the differences between these attitudes in order to comprehend what it is we truly believe in how we live our lives.

I hear these three words conflict with each other on a daily basis. I am convinced that, for one reason or another, society is or has become inherently negative toward any given situation; thus we convince ourselves that what may be difficult yet possible is not possible at all. I argue that this inherently negative outlook holds us back from pursuing and experiencing a genuinely happy life. I want to address this fact by looking at these three words individually: optimism, pessimism, and realism.

Optimism is defined as "a disposition or tendency to look on the more favorable side of events or conditions and to expect the most favorable outcome." Notice it is not defined as "a disposition or tendency to look on the more than favorable side of events or conditions and to expect the more than favorable outcome." I think people know what optimism means, but they choose to accept the latter definition as the true meaning. In other words, society views optimism as a "head-in-the-clouds" mindset, expecting the impossible.

Pessimism is defined as "a tendency to stress the negative or unfavorable or to take the gloomiest possible view." In this case, I believe people understand and accept this definition to be true. They think it is much more feasible to expect the worst possible outcome rather than the best possible outcome. However, whereas they do not accept a best possible outcome (as in optimism), they do accept the worst impossible outcome.

Realism is defined as an "interest in or concern for the actual or real, as distinguished from the abstract, speculative, etc." "Realism" suggests that we know what is real; but, as I will discuss later in the chapter called "Reality Is What You Make It", what is real is specific to each person. In short, our experiences shape our perspective of reality. So, if what is real is debatable, acting or being realistic is a fruitless debate. For example, it is likely a very real possibility for a Kennedy descendant to think they could have a successful career in politics. However, such a career will more than likely seem out of reach in the mind of a teen living on the streets of skid-row.

My goal is not to turn this book into a bunch of philosophical gibberish. Rather, I want you to ask yourself which frame of mind is most reasonable; optimism, pessimism, or realism?

We have already found that realism isn't rational because what is real or possible is dependent on the person. So, that leaves optimism and pessimism. What do people with either mindset typically say? The optimist says something like, "I may not have the experience, the money, or know the right people to start the next Microsoft, but I know I can do it." The pessimistic person says something like, "I really want to create the next Microsoft, but I'm not in that circle of rich people. It wouldn't matter if I had all the experience, money, or people on my side anyhow. It's just not possible."

Is the optimistic person being unreasonable? Are their dreams just too big? Obviously not. The optimist knows that they will have to work hard and sacrifice a lot to make their dream possible, but that dream is indeed possible. The dream was possible for Bill Gates (Microsoft), Michael Dell (Dell Computers), Howard Schultz (Starbucks); why not you? The world is full of people willing to tell you why software will never amount to anything, that computers will never be personal or used in the home, or that nobody in their right mind will pay $4 for a cup of coffee.

Is the pessimistic person being so irrational that what they spout as common sense is actually nonsensical? Clearly. Massive successes have happened in the past, are happening right now, and will undoubtedly happen again for as long as we are on this earth. To say "it's just not possible" is to say that there will never be another successful business. The pessimist wants us to believe that they are preaching responsibility and rationality when they are actually being the least rational of all. They are accepting the worst impossible outcome.

I have just briefly debunked realism and pessimism as acceptable mindsets. Yes, I am saying that we should all be the über optimist. I am saying that it only makes sense to not just hope for the best possible outcome but to expect the best because the optimist inherently understands that even if the best outcome is not achieved, what is likely to be accomplished will be greater than most would deem possible.

So what does this all boil down to? I have no doubt that every single person can achieve happiness in their life. It is not determined by the cards life has dealt you. People all too often say

Optimism, Pessimism, Realism

they would be happy if it wasn't for... No. Achieving happiness in life is accomplished by choosing the only rational mindset (optimism) and by choosing to make a great day.

In the next chapter I will explain what it is to make a great day and introduce you to a truly remarkable man; Frosty Westering. In my opinion, this next chapter is the most important of this entire book. It delves into how I choose to live my life now that I have survived cancer and how I hope you choose to live your life from now on. I promise you will live a life you only dreamed possible and those around you will notice a significant change about you that they would like to see in themselves, if you choose to make a great day.

3. *Make A Great Day*

My senior year at George R. Curtis Senior High School I took a day off of school to tour the campus of Pacific Lutheran University and to have a meeting with Coach Frosty Westering about playing collegiate football. The moment I met this man I couldn't help but love him. I knew I was in the presence of greatness. His character dripped with compassion and unconditional love for all people. Our meeting, surprisingly to me, had very little to do with football, but revolved around the subject of life, being an outstanding member of society, and being a model student athlete. Unfortunately, I later found torn ligaments in my right wrist from the previous football season which ended my time on the field before it began. Although I did not end up playing football at PLU, meeting Frosty left an impact upon me I wouldn't appreciate fully until I was diagnosed with cancer.

I had known about his book, "Make the Big Time Where You Are", for several years, but meeting him encouraged me to read it. The central message of the book is that life is going to happen whether you are ready or not; whether you want it to or not. There is no point in waiting to become great when you can be as great as you can currently be right now. A corresponding quote Frosty is known for is, "Make a great day!"

At first, this sounds like a cute play off of the common, "Have a great day." But if you study the phrase you will learn it is so much more. To have a great day assumes that a great day will come to you regardless of any effort you may or may not put forth. To make a great day tells one that in order to guarantee a great day of happening, we must actively pursue it rather than expect it to come to us. If there is one thing you take with you from reading this book, let this be it.

What will happen if you choose not to make a great day? Let's say you blow this chapter off as stupid motivational garbage. What will happen? Simple. The life you live will not change. Your life will not change either for the better or for the worse; you'll simply continue living your existence as you have known it.

We are all witnesses as to what the "have a great day" life is like since we are unable to recognize and make the change until a certain amount of maturity has been built. The have-a-great-day-ers complain about their work, their relationships, their this, and their that. These people complain about anything and everything because they are waiting for good things to happen. They feel they deserve good to happen to them because they have been waiting for so long. However, they refuse to see the good that is right in front of them. They are waiting to "have a great day."

It is really easy to spot a have-a-great-day-er; almost everybody is one. To "make a great day" is not a new concept, but one that we have a hard time accepting and incorporating into our daily lives. For some reason it is much easier to complain and to think negatively than it is to be positive. Just look back at how we view the words optimism, pessimism, and realism. Have you ever tried to look at a stranger and find three good things you like about them? Chances are that you will have a list of things you don't like before you even start! The same is true for your everyday acquaintances. If you were asked, "Tell me three things about your coworker Brittany," chances are you will think first about how loud she is when on the phone, the annoying sounds she makes when snaking at her desk, and how ugly her dress was at the latest company party before you acknowledge her great leadership abilities. I am by no means a psychological expert, but I'm willing to bet that we all do this because we want to see ourselves as superior to others, even if we have exceptional self-esteem.

What will happen if you do choose to make a great day? If you do decide to make your days great, you will still complain; only not as much and you will catch yourself when you do. I know you were hoping I would say, "You will no longer complain! You will only see the good in things! Your life will be nothing but perfect! You will be able to turn stone into gold!" But, seriously, we are only human.

● ● ●

Make A Great Day

If you decide to be a make-a-great-day-er, you will continue to be human and make the same mistakes we all make. However, the difference between making the switch and not is recognizing when we are being less than positive, evaluating the situation, and changing it for the better. The most interesting thing about these two groups of people is that the largest differentiator between them is exceptionally small; the will to recognize when their attitude is unproductive and deciding to change it for the better.

I think an example is needed to better illustrate the difference of a have-a-great-day-er and a make-a-great-day-er. Here's the situation: Let's say you are working in a dead end job. There is no chance for advancement, you live paycheck to paycheck, and the people you work with annoy you to high heaven. (This example is easy for me to put together because I have been in this precise position.) The have-a-great-day-er would bitch and moan about every detail about the job, dwell on what others are doing, and stick with the job because there is nothing else they can do. In their mind they are stuck; they are waiting to "have a great day".

On the other hand, the make-a-great-day-er will acknowledge that there are aspects of the job which they do not like; however, they make the choice to not dwell on the negative, but seek a positive. The make-a-great-day-er may say, "True, there are a lot of things I don't like about this job, but you know what? I am a people person, and I really do enjoy working with the customers." The make-a-great-day-er did not lie to themselves by saying, "I love this job… I love this job… I love this job!" Instead, they faced reality but found good in the bad. If they were unable to find any good, they would actually be a have-a-great-day-er masquerading as a make-a-great-day-er. This isn't necessarily a bad thing; only, a better understanding of what it means to "make a great day" is needed. A next step may be to take matters into their own hands and look for work they will enjoy more. Sometimes it is simply not enough to search for the good in the bad. Sometimes we need to acknowledge an even greater good (our personal satisfaction) and, in this case, find a different job.

     In retrospect, I realize that when I was diagnosed with my cancer I miraculously made the leap from being a have-a-great-day-er to being a make-a-great-day-er. I honestly do not know how or precisely when the change occurred. I suppose the initial shock of the diagnosis could have pushed the psychological button that needed to be pushed for me to become a make-a-great-day-er. It is absolutely fascinating how being forced to contemplate your own mortality can change your entire perception of life.

     The night I was diagnosed was when I first realized something had changed within me. I met my best friend, Marisa, on the waterfront in Ruston (a suburb of Tacoma) and sat on a dock where I told her the news of my diagnosis. "It's just not fair" she said. "Why does somebody as nice and caring as you have to get cancer? You're a good person. You don't deserve this." Without a thought I replied, "Just think of it this way. For some reason God needed to give somebody cancer; like there's some sort of quota that needs to be filled. I'm just happy He gave it to me because I know I'm strong enough to beat it. The way I see it, I'm saving someone's life." I didn't know it then, but I was already a make-a-great-day-er. I found the good in the tragic. I decided to make it a great cancer.

     Although I am no longer undergoing treatment, I continue to be a make-a-great-day-er. Perhaps it is a bit easier for me to adopt this lifestyle because I did face a life threatening illness. But that stage of my life is over now. I survived, and I have moved on, but I refuse to forget the lesson learned about making a great day. I often say, "Cancer is the best thing to have ever happened to me. Regardless of what is going on in my life, no matter what the weather is like, I wake up every day, look up to the sky and smile. It is a great day, no matter what. It is a great day because there was a time I didn't know if I would see the next day. It is a great day because I am alive and life is wonderful." And that is something

Make A Great Day

we can all agree on. Every day is a great day because I am alive to enjoy it.

4.   *Reality Is What You Make It*

I have struggled for quite some time trying to find the right words to describe what I have learned since my diagnosis. In my own mind I know exactly what I have discovered and I apply it every day of my now amazingly wonderful life. But, when it came to putting this newfound knowledge on paper, I was stumped. No matter how hard I tried, what I wrote didn't clearly or accurately communicate what I want to relay to you the reader. That was until I took a break from writing and read a series of books famously known as Rich Dad, Poor Dad written by Robert T. Kiyosaki.

In his series of books, Robert Kiyosaki tells the stories of his biological father (his "Poor Dad") who successfully climbed the ladder of the state educational system in Hawai'i and of his best friend's father (his "Rich Dad") who became one of the richest men in the state of Hawai'i. He referred to his real father as "Poor Dad" because despite becoming a successful educator and making more and more money throughout his career, his expenses grew with his income which forced him to always worry about being able to cover his financial liabilities. He referred to his best friend's father as "Rich Dad" because although he was unemployed, this man created businesses which grew to more than pay for his expenses. Yes, these books are about becoming financially independent and not necessarily about living a happy life in the context in which I write. However, the underlying message in the books is precisely what I want to convey: reality is what we make it.

Kiyosaki explains that the reason his Poor Dad stayed "poor" was because he lived by the popular notion that you should do well in school, so you can get in to a good college, so you can get a good job with a good retirement package. He believed that there was a scarce amount of money in the world, and this was the best way to live a comfortable life. Conversely, he explains that his Rich Dad was rich because he lived by the unpopular notion that you should do well in school, so you can get in to a good college, so you can create your own business(es) and make enough money to comfortably support your family for several generations. He believed that the world had limitless amounts of money, and this was the best way to live a comfortable life. Two very conflicting perspectives.

The two men wanted the same thing in the end; a comfortable life. However, Poor Dad's reality was that the world had a limited amount of money whereas Rich Dad's reality was that there was enough money in the world for anybody to get as much of it as they could imagine. In other words, they both got what they believed, but only one of them got what they wanted. Their reality was what they made it.

I believe the world is a pleasant place, people are intrinsically good, and every cloud has a silver lining. This can be admittedly difficult to assume when we watch the news every day and see gang shootings, terrorist attacks on a seemingly daily basis, and politicians spending their time fighting instead of working together for the common good. Be that as it may, I strive to find good/positivity in the seemingly bad/negativity every day. It is because I believe the world is a good place that I live a happy life. It is because I say that I will lead a happy life that I have a happy life. Life is great because I say it is.

I live this philosophy in every aspect of my life from the most significant of events to the seemingly insignificant. For example, as I am writing this book the world is experiencing an economic catastrophe and I am a direct result of its mercilessness. In February of 2009 I was laid off of my job as a corporate consultant for the most prestigious consulting firm in the world. I planned to build a solid career there and use that experience to be set for life. But, for the last ten months I have been living off of my unemployment insurance, which barely covers my monthly living expenses, and it looks like there is little likelihood of things to change in the near future.

Instead of bitching and moaning about my misfortune, complaining about my company's decision to lay me off, and wallowing in a pool of my own misery, my mindset has unwaveringly been, "This is just another opportunity to grow as a person and it will eventually open career and life doors I had not expected." Notice that I say that this is an opportunity. Calling this an opportunity is me choosing to make reality what I want it to be. This is an example of what is most certainly a significant life experience. (Update: Since I wrote this, I have since accepted a position at another consulting firm where I am much happier, and brought me home to Seattle from Los Angeles. Life has a way of rewarding those who see its merits.)

An example of when I use the same mindset in an insignificant instance is when I stub my toe. Don't laugh. I'm serious. I have been known to be a bit clumsy at times and I have the tendency to stub my toe quite often (maybe I should cut back on wearing sandals all the time). We all know what it is like to get that sudden shock of pain. We typically scream, cry, curse, etc. But when I hurt myself like that, you'll see me take in a big, deep breath and let it out slowly as I say either internally or externally, "Ok, that hurt. But it's not as bad as it could have been. It's not like going through chemo." I then walk it off and it is hardly an issue thereafter. I make a startling and perhaps excruciating experience less so by telling myself it's not so bad. I make my reality what I want it to be: less painful. Sure, I think that things become less painful the more you experience painful things or if you have experienced something much more painful, but that's beside the point.

There is absolutely no reason whatsoever that you cannot live as I do. There is no reason you cannot have a happy life simply by deciding to do so. All it takes is the decision to go against the grain, to live life contrary to the way most believe it should be lived. When I look around and notice that the vast majority of people are not very happy, or not as pleased with their life as they could be, it amazes me as to how hard a choice this decision is for most people to make. Perhaps people do not view it as a choice, but as fact. That is a cop out, not wanting to make the effort of making a better reality.

• • •

Reality Is What You Make It

Robert Kiyosaki (and his wife) is a product of the mindset he adopted. He and his wife were living out of their car when they decided they wanted to retire in ten years from that date; a pretty tall order. "Impossible!" most would say. They retired in nine. Regardless if you are interested in personal finance and becoming financially free or not, I strongly recommend reading the Rich Dad, Poor Dad book series. Each book delves into making your own reality and is therefore very pertinent to what I am advocating here. My favorite of the series (and in my opinion the most inspirational) is Retire Young, Retire Rich by Robert Kiyosaki. Kiyosaki discusses the leverage of your mind, the leverage of your plan, and the leverage of your actions; all important in making your own reality. Remember, the book is written in reference to making money; however, I the content is 100% applicable to living a happy life.

5.   *Is It Possible To Be Happy All The Time?*

I would be surprised if you haven't already been thinking, "Damn it Brad, what you are saying just isn't reasonable! You expect everybody to be happy and positive all the time? How is that possible?" Well, I'd be lying if I said the same thoughts haven't flown through my mind. I have to confess that despite learning all I have from having had cancer, I have been frustrated and saddened from time to time. Sometimes more than others. When these feelings occur I begin to consider myself hypocritical that I am writing this book yet I am not able to follow my own advice.

After all, my purpose for writing this second half of the book is to share what I have learned in hopes that others will be so overwhelmed by my happiness in life that they will strive to live in line with what I am preaching. If there are times when I can't help but feel the opposite of what I believe, how can I ask others to conform to my ideal?

I have battled with myself about this constantly and I have come to a fairly simple and obvious conclusion: we are not able to comprehend happiness unless we also experience sadness. That is true for anything in life. How can one know what it is like to be rich unless they have once had to struggle to get by? How can one feel tired if they have never been energetic? How can one be in love if they have never seen or felt love? How can one feel ill if they have never been healthy? To be able to have any feeling, we must also understand the opposite of that feeling.

So here is the answer to our question: No. We can never be happy all the time. And thank God for that! If we never have moments of sadness we can never be happy. If we never felt sadness we would forever wonder what else we could feel. We would ask ourselves, "Is there more to life? Is this really all I have to live for? What do they have that I don't?" Without sadness we would be in an endless state of contentment; never expecting more or less because we would not know it exists. That is pretty

● ● ●

upsetting if you really think about it. Imagine, we would likely all be extremely depressed if were in a constant state of happiness. We wouldn't know to appreciate that happiness and might ask ourselves why we never feel better than that!

Prior to my diagnosis I took life for granted because I had never been faced with the very real possibility of death. I now respect and cherish life because I do know what it is like to face death. Unfortunately, most people do not recognize the opportunity or face a stimulus to appreciate life; and, if they do, it is commonly at an old age with much of their life already behind them. Most people go through life saying they love life while they continue to complain about the weather, gossip about others, have road rage, and wait to have a good day. As I have said before, cancer is the best thing to have ever happened to me. If I were given the choice to never have had cancer and not know what I know now, or have cancer again and not know the outcome, I would choose to face cancer again. The education the disease has bestowed me is truly priceless.

So, if we cannot expect (or truly want) to be happy all the time, what is to be said about those times when we are depressed, impatient, frustrated? I continue to learn that what we must do when we are faced with these unpleasant times is to first admit that this is only temporary and is necessary for us to have more uplifting feelings later on. Next, we need to try and understand why it is we feel the way we do. It is too easy to tell ourselves we are pissed off simply because we are pissed off. We rarely take the time to try and understand the basis for our feelings; rather, we simply ride them off as something we are feeling for the time being without any justification. The truth is we feel for a reason. We get butterflies in our stomach with a first kiss because we are excited. We get angry when friends don't support us because we feel betrayed. We are nervous at a job interview because we do not want to screw up the opportunity. If we refuse to try and understand the reasons behind our feelings we cannot begin to address those feelings. The longer we wait, the longer we will feel pain and therefore we will experience less happiness.

Once we allow ourselves to understand our feelings, we can then begin to act upon them and face the issue at hand. What I mean by "face the issue at hand" is to ask the question, "Now that I know why I am feeling this way, what do I need to change it? What do I need to do to be happy?" It is a simple question, but a pivotal step in making a great day.

We are the only one who can truthfully answer this question; unless, that is, if the reason for what we feel is so ambivalent that it requires the assistance of a therapist. I believe that since we are the ones that understand why we are feeling the way we do, we are the ones who ultimately know how to go about changing the way we feel. I mention the assistance of a therapist for major issues because it is their job to first understand who we are from an unbiased perspective and to then help point us in the right direction for us to solve our problems. I view a therapist as an extension of us. I do not think they have the answers to our problems; rather, they have the ability to see through the clutter of our own mind and aid us in finding what we already know but are not able to understand.

I feel it necessary to make a brief side note. Society has manipulated the purpose of therapy to be for drastically mentally ill people who are overemotional, incompetent, or for one reason or another "crazy". It is sad to see how we have stigmatized this profession; this very needed service. In my very humble opinion, everybody should go to a therapist. Of course, some require more visits more than others, but I view therapy like an oil change for your car; it's something you need to do to keep the engine running smoothly. Sure, you can refuse to change your oil, but after a while you're going to a lot of issues that could have been easily prevented. Ok, that tangent is over, I promise.

Now that I've explained how I have found we can change our negative feelings into positive ones, I feel it necessary to also discuss a phrase we are all familiar with which typically refers to times when our feelings have been tried: "Forgive and forget".

6.　Never Forgive and Forget

How often do we hear the phrase "forgive and forget"? It has become more of an accepted cliché than a piece of advice. When listening to our friends' problems or overhearing an argument of a passing couple we almost certainly hear at least some variation of this saying. It is so widely accepted you would think it is its own amendment to the United States Constitution.

I used to agree with this saying. I used to think that to forgive and forget meant being the bigger and better person. After all, it is admirable to see somebody who is able to forgive their enemy as well as put their conflict so far behind them that it no longer affects them or their relationship. For example, on May 13th, 1981, Turkish extremist Mehmet Ali Agca attempted to assassinate Pope John Paul II by shooting him in St. Peter's Square. Later, in 1983, the Pope visited his would be assassin in his prison to forgive him. Not only that, but by request of the Pope, Agca was released from prison and extradited back to Turkey to serve time for another crime. In other words, Pope John Paul II forgave his would be assassin and chose to "forget" the incident evidenced by Agca's release from prison. Certainly, we would all like to view ourselves as so saintly.

Although "forgive and forget" is a widely held value, my battle with cancer has convinced me to think otherwise. I certainly agree that forgiveness is a necessary practice in leading a virtuous and happy life. However, opting to forget is choosing to be complacent and not better one's self.

I like to say that we are reflections of our experiences. What I mean is that our character is shaped by what we experience in life, and what we learn from those events is expressed through who we become as people, our character. As children we learned to raise our hand in the classroom when we have a question. In our careers we learn the culture and politics in our work environments so we know how to go about getting what we want. As adults we learn how to file our taxes appropriately so we won't get audited by the IRS. Everything we do in life is a result of learning from our previous experiences. Why then would we expect to benefit by following the popular adage of "forgive and forget"? The fact is we won't.

I mentioned it was my battle with cancer that shaped this belief of mine. Thankfully, I chose to maintain a positive perspective throughout my treatment. That isn't to say I didn't have absolute hatred for the potentially fatal invading disease in my body. Every day I was forced to face my cancer and there was no way I would embrace it with love and affection. Rather, I chose to express my hate for my cancer by keeping a positive attitude and kill it through determination (in addition to the chemotherapy). I learned more about myself each day, after each puking episode, after each wild emotional swing. Had I chosen to forgive and forget I would not be the person I am today.

If I chose to forgive and forget I would have accepted my cancer (which I did the moment I was diagnosed) but fail to learn anything from my journey. That is like graduating from four years of college with honors and immediately experiencing a brain injury that completely wipes out all the knowledge you paid for and work so hard to gain.

Who would I be today if I chose to forgive and forget my cancer? I would be the same person I was before July 30th, 2004. I would still be a determined person with a passion for excellence and success because I was very much that person before my cancer. However, I would more than likely face the world with a less than positive attitude, continue to blame others/other factors for any bad things that happen to me, take my friendships and other relationships for granted, see the glass half empty rather than half full… you get the picture.

I chose to forgive and remember. To forgive and remember is to accept what life throws at you and to use those experiences to make you a better person. Remembering my cancer has been the best decision I have ever made. Remembering my cancer has prompted me to co-direct the first annual Relay for Life at my college, Pacific Lutheran University. The year I helped begin

● ● ●

that annual event on campus we raised $42,000; $12,000 more than our goal of $30,000. I am happy to know that because I decided to remember my cancer I am in some way (regardless of how small) responsible for the funds that have been and will be raised in subsequent years.

Remembering my cancer encouraged me apply for an internship at the Lance Armstrong Foundation. As I explained earlier, my work at the LAF helped promote the foundation, improve the internal operations, and encourage others to raise funds. Who knows how much money my efforts indirectly raised?

Remembering my cancer has convinced me to position myself as a cancer advocate. Speaking to high schools, colleges, and communities has put my story in the ears of numerous people. I have heard from some people that my story motivated them to get checked out by their doctors when they noticed something they would have otherwise passed off as nothing to worry about. Perhaps remembering my cancer saved them (or will save them down the road) from having to face many of the horrendous things I had to endure.

Personally, remembering my cancer has built and reinforced many relationships. Doing so has created friendships that may otherwise not have been formed and has made me a better friend. I will say again that I now take my relationships with my family, friends, and others much less for granted. I know how important people are in our lives and I strive to relish in each moment I have these people. My relationship with life in general is perhaps the most improved since I have been faced with my own mortality, and doing so has taught me to be much more appreciative of all things.

These are just a few examples of how choosing to remember my cancer has shaped me into whom I am today. I make a point to learn not only from my cancer, but from everything life gives me. I choose to remember everything and forget nothing. I will never be perfect, but I know that I can continue to improve as long as there is air in my lungs and a spirit in my body. I feel that I owe it to God and to those who have not

● ● ●

been given a second chance at life to continuously improve myself. If I refuse to do so, this second chance at life will be wasted on somebody who doesn't appreciate it.

7.   *90% of Every Battle Is Mental*

In saying that cancer is the best thing to have ever happened to me, I have gotten a bit of pushback from what I am about to discuss. I am a firm believer that 90% of every battle is mental. The other 10% is up to a higher power, be it fate, God, whatever.

Remember when I was given a 50% chance of being cured? Dr. Senecal told me that I needed a fourth round of chemo because there was still living cancer in my body, and that only 50% of those who need this fourth round are typically cured. When I got that news, my mind was in a fog for precisely two days. I walked around with my head hanging, not a thought in my mind, and I cared about absolutely nothing. I felt lost.

For those two days I was zombie-like. I was mentally gone because all I could focus on was that there was a 50% chance that the cancer was going to kill me. However, on that second day, I was sitting in the Head Coach's office in the Curtis High School locker room before football practice when one of the fellow coaches (noticing my lifelessness) asked if I was feeling alright. I told the coaching staff the news I received the previous day and there wasn't any response. Just some "humms" and "uh-huhs". What can you tell a guy who just got such bad news?

I sat in that chair when what felt like some kind of revelation hit me. "Yeah, I have a 50% chance of dying" I told myself, "but I also have a 50% chance of surviving!" It may sound simple enough, but at that moment I no longer felt like I was going to die. I was suddenly filled with life and excitement.

"I may have a coin flip chance of surviving," I thought, "but (and pardon my French) fuck that! I'm going to put that coin flip on my side. I'm going to give myself a 51% chance of surviving by being positive! I've been positive up to this point, let's keep it up!"

I completely dismissed those two days of hell I put myself through because I knew right then and there that I was indeed

● ● ●

going to live through this thing. There was nothing anybody could say or do to convince me otherwise. If I was indifferent about my treatment I had a 50% chance of living or dying. But, if I kept positive, I would have a 51% chance of living. It was as simple as that.

I think I know what you are thinking to yourself right now. "That's a bunch of BS! Be positive and you can do whatever you want. Ha! What a bunch of crap!"

If that's what you're thinking, I'm honestly not surprised. It sounds like what many of our parents said to try and build self-esteem, "You can do anything you want in life if you put your mind to it." Be that as it may, that is exactly what I believe, no matter how corny it may sound.

Referring back once again to the chapter entitled "Pessimism, Optimism, Realism", we tend to think negatively rather than positively. We tend to think of why we can't rather than why we can. I think that, for the most part, I have control over what happens to me; that I am responsible for my future. Psychologists call this an internal locus of control. If you tend to believe that you do not have control over your future (that you simply have to play the hand life has dealt you) the first thing you need to do is learn to take control of your life. Refusing to do so will handicap you by placing any coin flip in your life against you. You will be giving yourself a 51% chance of failing.

I say 90% of every battle is mental. By being positive I did everything in my power to bring about my desired result; to survive. In other words, I believe that staying positive regardless of what life throws at you will result in achieving what you want 9 out of 10 times. If I accepted my bad news as a 50% chance of dying, I would then be relying on that remaining 10% to save my life. I'd rather have a 90% chance of living than a 10% chance.

I refer to the remaining 10% as "fate, God, whatever." This remaining 10% is completely out of your control. If you are a spiritual person you may believe that the world has a plan and your plan simply does not fit, and that is the reason for your failure. If you are a religious person you may believe that God or Allah has a plan and your plan doesn't fit with theirs, thus the reason for your failure. Perhaps the stars are not aligned properly, or karma is paying you a visit. Whatever your belief, we have the ability to determine our course in life up to the point where this higher power disagrees.

We have a duty as people to never give up on life. We must pursue survival when our lives are threatened. And, as was the case with my survival, I pursued survival by refusing to accept negativity and I willed myself to survive. I was positive. I am living proof that an optimistic outlook can allow you to determine your future. Unfortunately, there are plenty of people in the world who also prove that a negative outlook can do the same.

I have gotten a few very defensive reactions to this argument. Some people think that I believe if their loved one died, or they didn't get the promotion, or (fill in the blank), it was because they weren't positive enough, or they didn't want it hard enough. This is not at all what I am saying. I feel for those who have lost people they love to cancer and I am in no way insensitive enough to suggest that they died because they were not as positive as me. Unfortunately, I have to accept that regardless of how optimistic we may be, that remaining 10% does remain a factor. I believe things happen for a reason. I believe I survived because I kept optimism on my side and because God has a plan for me. I do not know why sometimes the most optimistic people still don't make it. Maybe they die because their memory makes us better people. I don't know. All I know is that things happen for a reason and all we can ask of ourselves is to do what is within our control; maintain a positive attitude, and fight to survive.

8.   *How Much Is Too Much?*

On three occasions since overcoming my bout with cancer, friends have confronted me regarding observations of theirs which forced me to ask myself some very serious questions. These friends revealed to me that, at times, they do not like the person I have become. The points they have put forth have forced me to question the person I have become and the ideals I have adopted at the core of my being. Needless to say, doing so has been very difficult as well as enlightening.

One of the concerns mentioned to me was when I was still in college. A small group of friends made their peace in several different ways, but the main complaint sounded something like this: "You bombard people with your cancer. Even if you don't know them, it seems the first thing you tell them is that you are a cancer survivor. You sound arrogant!"

When I first heard this I laughed it off thinking they were overreacting and just trying to piss me off a little. But, as time went by, I paid special close attention to the direction my conversations went whether I knew the person or not. I eventually realized that my friends weren't necessarily exaggerating. I noticed that I would often introduce my cancer to somebody rather than introduce myself.

Now, I wouldn't go up to somebody and say, "Hey, I'm Brad. I'm a cancer survivor," but I would manage to find a way to bring up my survivorship early in the conversation. When I observed this in myself I was immediately embarrassed. I couldn't believe I would try and upstage like this; it was so out of character. I am not one to crave attention. I love being active and striving for success, but the attention I often to renounce. It was then clear to me why my friends often thought the new people I met perceived me as an arrogant person.

Before I recognized this, I tried to explain to my friends that they simply did not understand what it felt like to overcome cancer. I would try and explain the feelings that overwhelmed me,

• • •

but I knew it was useless. It's just one of those things you can't understand unless you experience it first-hand. "I'm a different person now" I would say. "I am a survivor and I don't know how to be anything else." Finally, when I began to realize how "in your face" I was being, I made a point to bring it back a bit (well, more than a bit) and make sure people saw who I am rather than what I've gone through.

Don't get me wrong, my cancer does come up quite a bit, but it typically is brought up by the other person in a conversation. I wear five yellow LIVESTRONG bands on my right wrist (one for each person I know with cancer) and it is not uncommon for somebody to ask me why I wear so many. I explain I wear one for each person I know with cancer. I may then continue and say that I have one band tattooed on my right shoulder for myself, and I then show them my tattoo. My tattoo is of a wooden Celtic cross with "LIVESTRONG" inscribed on the cross bar of the cross. Also, a LIVESTRONG band stands in place of the cross's "halo". Finally, the date of my diagnosis and curing surgery are placed above and below the cross respectively. Between my wristbands and my tattoo, my cancer is brought up somewhat often.

The second observation that has been brought to my attention continues to bother me as I write this. The observations made by several friends can be summed up in a single phrase: "All you are is cancer!"

When I ask my friends what they mean by this, they tell me they get sick of hearing me speak so positively, compare things to what I experienced when going through chemo, watching me write this book, and coming into my condo and seeing the framed shadow box given to me by my parents which contains a hand written letter from Lance Armstrong wishing me well, a copy of his book, some pictures, a LIVESTRONG bracelet, and other such items. They argue that my entire life revolves around cancer and I do not allow for anything else. This is an argument I have not come to agree with, nor do I imagine myself coming to do so.

Let's look at their complaint. First, they are tired of hearing me speak so positively. Hearing this makes me sad not

• • •

only for them, but for the majority of people because I think the majority agrees with them. This complaint reinforces the arguments made in the chapter Optimism, Pessimism, Realism where I explain how people tend to be innately negative; even to the point where it makes little sense. I have carefully listened to the arguments friends have made about my "intensely optimistic" manner, but I have decided I simply do not agree. I agree to disagree.

On the other hand I do sympathize with them when they complain that I compare things too often to my cancer. I do not want to hear somebody tell the same story over and over again, so for that reason I agree that at times I can refer to my cancer too often. To be respectful of that, I pay careful attention to whom I am around when in a conversation. If something is being discussed where I think a comparison to my cancer experience would be appropriate, I try to respect who is around and only contribute in that manner if those around are not especially familiar with my story. If I feel it will be received well, I will go ahead and compare what we're talking about to my cancer.

I do not want to (nor will I) feel that I am always having to screen my conversations. I do, however, want to be respectful of those around and if they have heard me speak a lot about my cancer, I will either not say what is on my mind, or I will address it without reference to my cancer. However, at times I will deliberately mention my battle with cancer because I know my story is widely viewed as inspirational. If I can help somebody by telling my story, you better believe I will do so. There can be a fine line between being respectful for others and being respectful of the person(s) in need.

For the most part, people have been very supportive of my will to write this book. I explain that my motivation for writing is so my illness can serve as an aid for others going through similar events in their own life. People seem to respect that. However, there have been a select few that have accused me of only wanting to make money from the book, simply seeking fame/recognition, or of building a shrine to myself in the form of a book. Nothing could be further from the truth.

As I am writing this book, I have yet to seek out publishers. It is very likely that when I complete this book nobody will want to publish it. There is no promise of money in any way. Sure, I would love to make some money from it if it works out that way, but it is not my motivation. I have mentioned a few times throughout the book that I am not one to crave the lime light, so fame is clearly not of any interest. The same is the case for "building a shrine to myself" as well. I consider myself fairly selfless and take pride in that. I have no use for self-glorification.

An important concept for people to grasp is that from the day I was diagnosed I inherited a brand new family; the cancer community. I share a bond with millions of people around the world (1.5 million new people each year in the U.S.) that others simply do not understand. As a survivor, I feel a duty to those that have been, are, and will be survivors to help in ways I am able. I am writing this book for the sole purpose of helping my new family; people I know and people I do not know all over the world, yet love nonetheless.

Finally, a third complaint was brought to my intention. A friend of mine recently told me she didn't feel comfortable around me at times because I live as if cancer still resides in my body. "Between the shadow box in your condo, your tattoo, your LIVESTRONG bands, and the way you talk, it's like you still aren't cured of your cancer!" she said.

To be honest, I was quite taken aback by her comments because I thought I had been doing just fine since my college friends brought up similar concerns years earlier. I tried to explain that I hope to never be "over my cancer", meaning I do not want to forget what I have learned and resort back to taking life for granted. She and I talked about what she had to say and the conversation eventually ended because I was not able to clearly understand her stance. She admitted it is possible she just doesn't understand how I look at life because she has never been forced to contemplate her own mortality. In the end I promised to try and not speak about cancer around her. I did so because we are friends and I do not mind making small sacrifices out of respect for her and our friendship.

I have come to the conclusion that those who do not appreciate hearing my story or references to my story are uncomfortable because they either have been tragically affected by the disease or they know nothing about it and are scared of the unknown. That is certainly understandable and respectable. It is difficult at times because I feel that my cancer has opened my eyes to a lifetime worth of knowledge and insight and I want to better the lives of as many people I can by infecting them with what I have learned.

Many people are very receptive to what I have to say. Still, many others simply do not want to hear it. It pains me because those are the people that need help the most. Those are the ones that complain about everything and anything and hate the world for the hand it has dealt them. I watch them walk away and say to myself, "No! Come back! I can help make your life so much better!" I know I cannot help everybody, but that is little consolation when I see my pre-cancer self in them and they turn away. I am living proof that a good and happy life is chosen not received, and my greatest wish is to help these people see what I see now, and do so before they are forced to face their own death; before it is too late for them.

9.   *Conclusion*

I hope my story has provided insight to what you or your loved one may experience while battling this horrible disease we call cancer. You will inevitably experience many of the same events and emotions as I did. However, you will undoubtedly face obstacles which differ from mine. For that reason I strongly encourage you to share your story in whatever way(s) you are comfortable. You decided to read this book because you had questions and wanted to learn from my experience. Be that resource for others. When you are diagnosed with cancer, you become part of a family; a family of survivors. They need to learn from you. Just as you would be there for your mother, father, or siblings, be there for them by sharing your story.

I also hope that sharing what I have learned about life has been inspiring. I am all too aware that some of it sounds idealistic and impracticable. But I promise you, if you allow yourself to fully embrace what I have written you will live in a world few others do. Skies will seem clearer, pain will be deadened, relationships will be more fulfilling, and life will simply be all around better! Not only that, but you will no longer all self-imposed limitations prevent you from attaining your goals. Determine to be optimistic and make a great day, never forgive and forget, and put the odds in your favor by sustaining a positive attitude.

I will leave you with a quote I stumbled upon just as I am about to publish this book. It succinctly delivers the message I have tried to deliver throughout each and every page. Thank you for reading. I wish you a lifetime of health and happiness.

I would rather be ashes than dust!
I would rather that my spark should burn out in a brilliant blaze
than it should be stifled by dry-rot.
I would rather be a superb meteor, every atom of me in
magnificent glow, than a sleepy and permanent planet.
The proper function of man is to live, not to exist.
I shall not waste my days in trying to prolong them.
I shall use my time.

~Jack London
Jack London's Tales of Adventure
(New York: Doubleday, 1956), p. vii